Aesthetic Series
Hair Transplantation

Aesthetic Series
Hair Transplantation

Editors

Nicole Rogers MD FAAD
Assistant Clinical Professor
Tulane University School of Medicine
Department of Dermatology
Metairie, Louisiana, USA

Meena K Singh MD
Dermatologic Surgeon at
KMC Hair Center
Shawnee, KS
Overland Park
Kansas City, Missouri, USA

Shannon Watkins MD
Dermatologist
Mount Sinai Hospital
Department of Dermatology
New York, NY, USA

Series Editor

Marc R Avram MD
Clinical Professor of Dermatology
Department of Dermatology
Weill Cornell Medical College, New York
Presbyterian Hospital, New York, NY, USA

JAYPEE The Health Sciences Publisher
New Delhi | London | Philadelphia | Panama

Jaypee Brothers Medical Publishers (P) Ltd

Headquarters
Jaypee Brothers Medical Publishers (P) Ltd.
4838/24, Ansari Road, Daryaganj
New Delhi 110 002, India
Phone: +91-11-43574357
Fax: +91-11-43574314
E-mail: jaypee@jaypeebrothers.com

Overseas Offices
J.P. Medical Ltd.
83, Victoria Street, London
SW1H 0HW (UK)
Phone: +44-20 3170 8910
Fax: +44(0)20 3008 6180
E-mail: info@jpmedpub.com

Jaypee-Highlights Medical Publishers Inc.
City of Knowledge, Bld. 237, Clayton
Panama City, Panama
Phone: +1 507-301-0496
Fax: +1 507-301-0499
E-mail: cservice@jphmedical.com

Jaypee Medical Inc.
The Bourse
111 South Independence Mall East
Suite 835, Philadelphia, PA 19106, USA
Phone: +1 267-519-9789
E-mail: jpmed.us@gmail.com

Jaypee Brothers Medical Publishers (P) Ltd.
17/1-B, Babar Road, Block-B, Shaymali
Mohammadpur, Dhaka-1207
Bangladesh
Mobile: +08801912003485
E-mail: jaypeedhaka@gmail.com

Jaypee Brothers Medical Publishers (P) Ltd.
Bhotahity, Kathmandu, Nepal
Phone: +977-9741283608
E-mail: kathmandu@jaypeebrothers.com

Website: www.jaypeebrothers.com
Website: www.jaypeedigital.com

Inquiries for bulk sales may be solicited at: jaypee@jaypeebrothers.com

Aesthetic Series—Hair Transplantation

First Edition: **2016**

ISBN: 978-93-5152-932-3

Printed at: Ajanta Offset & Packagings Ltd., New Delhi

Dedicated to

All persons, both young and old, who are
thrilled by the magic of hair transplantation.

—Nicole Rogers

In memory of my father, Dr. Awadh Nath Singh;
and dedicated to my beautiful children, Anjali, Avani,
and Akari; my mother, Dr. Linda Singh; and my siblings,
Dr Sarita, Arjuna, Jaipal and Asha Singh.

—Meena K Singh

My mom, my dad, and my husband.
Thank you for all your love and support throughout
the years. You are the best. I love you!

—Shannon Watkins

My wife, Robin and two children Robert and Jacob
for their unconditional love and support each and every day.

My parents, Morrell and Maria Avram who have always
loved me, supported me, and for whom I am eternally grateful.

My brothers and sister, Joe, Louis, Eric, Mathew, David,
Harry, and Rella, for your love, friendship, and advice.

My coeditors, Nicole Rogers, Meena K Singh and
Shannon Watkins for teaching me so much over the years.

Michele Egan, Dayanna McLean,
Ellen Murphy-Smith for helping create an outstanding
team that cares about each of our patients.

—Marc R Avram

Contributors

Marc R Avram MD
Clinical Professor of Dermatology
Department of Dermatology
Weill Cornell Medical College
New York
Presbyterian Hospital
New York, NY, USA

Duane Dilworth MD
Dermatologist
Howard University
College of Medical
Washington DC, USA

Francisco Jimenez-Acosta MD FISHRS
Mediteknia Dermatology and
Hair Transplant Clinic
Las Palmas Gran Canaria
Canary Islands, Spain
Associate Researcher
Medical Pathology Group
University of Las Palmas de Gran
Canaria, Las Pahmas, Spain

Nicole Rogers MD FAAD
Assistant Clinical Professor
Tulane University School of
Medicine
Department of Dermatology
Metairie, Louisiana, USA

Meena K Singh MD
Dermatologic Surgeon at
KMC Hair Center
Shawnee, KS
Overland Park
Kansas City, Missouri, USA

Robin Unger MD
Assistant Professor
Department of Dermatology
Mount Sinai School of Medicine
New York, NY, USA

Shannon Watkins MD
Dermatologist
Mount Sinai Hospital
Department of Dermatology
New York, NY, USA

Carlos K Wesley MD
Private Practice
New York, NY, USA

Craig Ziering DO FAOCD
Director for the Hair Loss
Medicine & Surgery Fellowship
Southampton Hospital, New York
Assistant Clinical Professor
Dermatology and Surgery
University of California
Irvine School of Medicine
CEO/Medical Director
Ziering Medical Worldwide
World Headquarters
Los Angeles, California, USA

Foreword

Hair transplantation is a field as with all of medicine that has changed and evolved rapidly over the past several years. This book is dedicated to the latest techniques in the aesthetic and medical applications of hair transplant surgery. Today all patients should expect completely natural appearing transplanted hair and the reason is the exclusive use of follicular units in our patients. This book, which is a gathering of renowned colleagues from all over the world, we hope will help illustrate some of the techniques and advice to consistently achieve naturally appearing transplanted hair for our patients.

Marc R Avram MD
Clinical Professor of Dermatology
Department of Dermatology
Weill Cornell Medical College, New York
Presbyterian Hospital, New York, NY, USA

Preface

Hair transplantation as with all of medicine has evolved rapidly over the past several years. Currently, women and men can consistently expect natural appearing transplanted hair. This book reviews the latest techniques in the aesthetic and reconstructive hair transplant surgery. Each chapter is written by leading contributors in the innovations that have occurred in the procedure over the past several years.

The era of the follicular unit extraction has allowed patients to now undergo a hair transplant with minimal textural changes in their skin. This allows our patients to style their hair any way they desire with no scar ever evident. During the era of large graft surgery, women rarely benefited from the procedure. In the era of the follicular unit transplantation, millions of women have had a natural frame of hair restored to their face.

We hope this book will allow both the novice and experience hair transplant surgeons to benefit from the ideas throughout the book.

Nicole Rogers
Meena K Singh
Shannon Watkins

Acknowledgments

I would like to thank my coeditors, Nicole Rogers, Meena K Singh and Shannon Watkins for their hard work in helping create this book.

In addition, I would like to thank Michele Egan, Dayanna McLean, Ellen Murphy-Smith, and Elizabeth Murray for their contributions in making this book. Their efforts and ideas for patient care and how to perform the best hair transplant surgery possible for our patients is much appreciated and reflected in some of the ideas in this book.

I would like to thank our contributing authors who have dedicated their time to help share their knowledge, time and experience with others in order to improve the quality and care for patients. Many hours on your part was given to share your knowledge with others.

Finally, I would also like to thank Mr Jitendar P Vij (Group Chairman), Mr Ankit Vij (Group President) Ms Chetna Malhotra Vohra (Associate Director), Ms Angima Shree (Development Editor) and production team of Jaypee Brothers Medical Publishers (P) Ltd., New Delhi, India.

Contents

CHAPTER 1

The Consult

Meena K Singh

INTRODUCTION

The consult is paramount to the success of hair restoration surgery. Building a good patient–doctor interaction begins with the patient's initial encounters with the office. This initial aspect of the consultation may start with online research on the office website, an initial phone call, or any brochure or reading materials.

During the consultation, determination if the patient is a proper candidate will be established. In addition, the consultation is the opportunity to properly set patient expectations and review all of the details of the surgery, including any preoperative or postoperative care. If conducted well, the consultation alone can increase the patient's satisfaction with their own procedure. The consultation may be performed in combination with a designated consultant.

CANDIDATE SELECTION

Candidate selection is a major determinant of the success of the surgery. This process establishes if a patient is medically and psychologically appropriate for the procedure. Assessing criteria such as age, degree of hair loss, donor supply, hair caliber, and hair color will aid in selection. The proper candidate should have adequate donor supply to achieve coverage of the desired recipient areas, control of the ongoing hair loss, and most importantly, reasonable expectations.

Age

Individuals who are 25 and older are preferable for hair transplantation. The indefinite use of medication to slow ongoing hair loss cannot be assumed. Therefore, the rate and eventual severity of the hair loss are much less predictable in individuals younger than 25. Compared to older candidates, these younger patients are more likely to desire to return to their original versus a more mature hairline, which may not be a reasonable expectation.

Setting Realistic Expectations

Setting realistic expectations of the perceived density that can be achieved will dictate how satisfied the patient is with the final cosmetic outcome of the procedure. Hair restoration surgery is no longer the "hair plugs" of the past. There has been a significant shift from large, 10–25 follicular unit grafts to smaller, more naturally occurring one to three follicular unit grafts (Fig. 1.1). The goal is to improve the patients' appearance without being able to detect the performed surgery. The expected outcome of the hair transplant is a natural, undetectable improvement that should never look pluggy. Moreover, even with smaller, follicular unit grafts, the transplant can still look unnatural if the hairline is too straight and lacks irregularity. The final outcome of the hair transplant should mimic the "irregularly, irregular" appearance of naturally occurring hairlines (Fig. 1.2).

Importantly, the patient's primary area of cosmetic concern should be established. They may desire an enhanced hairline, reinforcement of the frontal scalp, and/or thickening of the vertex scalp (Fig. 1.3). The most cosmetically significant improvement is achieved by enhancing the hair that frames the face by reinforcing the frontotemporal

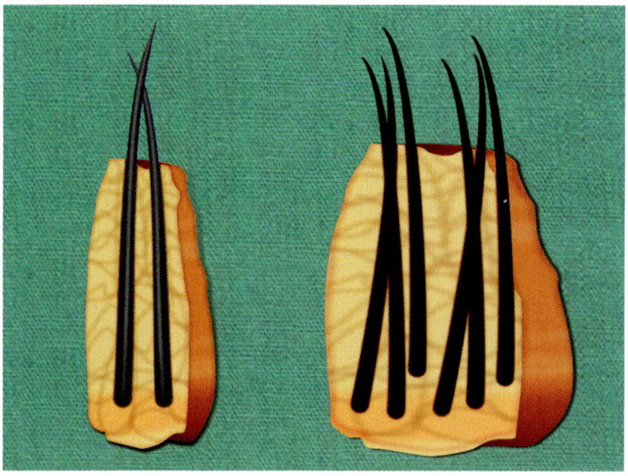

Fig. 1.1: With modern hair transplantation, smaller one to three follicular unit grafts are used (A) versus the larger "pluggy" grafts of the past.

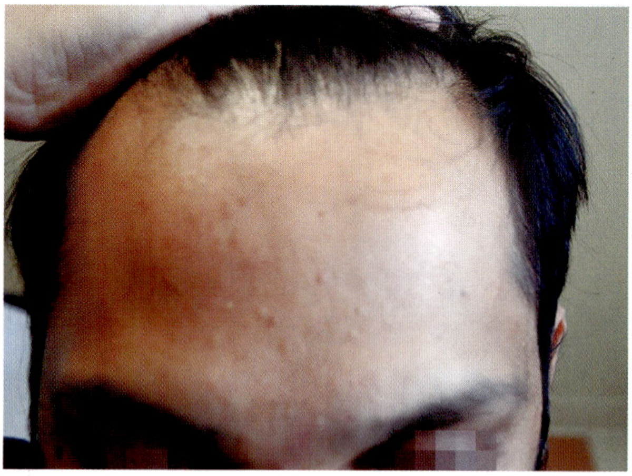

Fig. 1.2: Patient demonstrating a natural-appearing hairline.

hairline and increasing the perceived density of the frontal scalp. In addition, the hair transplant should be designed in anticipation of ongoing hair loss. This ensures that the outcome looks natural in the immediate as well as distant future. Therefore, if the patient has limited donor supply and a significant degree of balding, they should be counseled that the most significant cosmetic outcome will be achieved by mainly concentrating on the areas that frame the face. Explaining this concept is especially important to men with androgenetic alopecia who desire a lowered hairline and/or enhanced coverage of the vertex scalp. If grafts are placed too anteriorly and the hairline continues to recede, the patient will be left with rows of transplanted hairs unnaturally anterior to the receded frontal hairline. When counseling men who desire hair transplant of the vertex scalp, it should be explained that even if full coverage of the vertex scalp is achieved with the hair transplant, it may not be significantly noticeable to the patient. In addition, because the follicular whorl in the vertex scalp all lie in different directions, more grafts are needed to adequately cover this area. Moreover, if the ongoing hair loss is not controlled, the patient may be left with a highly unnatural-appearing ring of alopecia surrounding the grafts. Considering the long-term cosmetic result, transplanting follicular units in the frontal two-thirds of the scalp is the safest region.

Most importantly, the perceived density that can be achieved is a function of not only the density of transplanted grafts but also the hair wave and caliber.

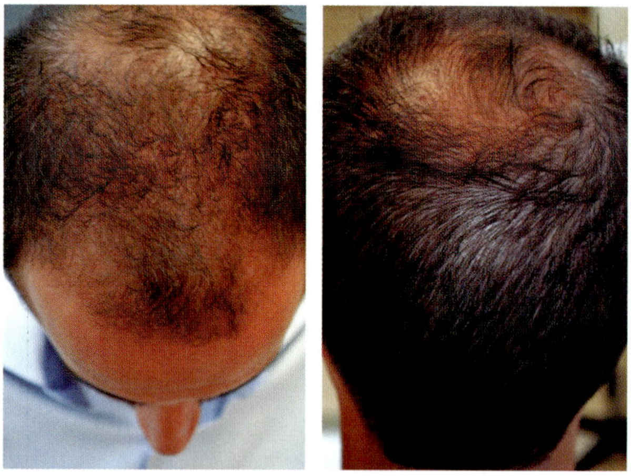

Fig. 1.3: A common consult. A 28-year-old man demonstrating a receding frontotemporal hairline and thinning in the frontal and vertex scalp.

A patient with thin, wispy hair should not expect the same cosmetic improvement as an individual with thick, curly hair. Even with the same number of grafts transplanted and equivalent growth, thick, curly hair can appear from 50% to 100% denser than fine, straight hair. Moreover, the net density is equivalent to the number of transplanted hairs minus any ongoing hair loss of the existing hairs in the recipient area. Creating a significantly perceptible net increase is more difficult in patients with rapid, ongoing hair loss compared to those with a slower hair loss rate or whose hair loss has been controlled medically (*see* Chapter 10).

Additional surgeries may be necessary to achieve the desired outcome. This may be a reflection of ongoing hair loss or any technical limitations in the primary surgery that prevented the full desired coverage. Depending on the size of the recipient areas, rate of ongoing hair loss, and donor supply, most can achieve the desired cosmetic goal within two surgeries.

Detailed History

Hair transplantation is one option for the treatment of alopecia; however, it may not be the optimal treatment for the patient. As with any hair loss evaluation, it is first necessary to obtain the proper diagnosis. Hair restoration surgery on types of alopecia other than androgenetic alopecia takes special considerations (*see* Chapter 8) and may have varied overall outcomes; therefore, it is important to be able to confidently identify androgenetic alopecia from potential scarring mimickers. This entails taking a detailed history (Table 1.1), performing a thorough scalp examination, and potentially doing further workup, such as obtaining a biopsy. Individuals with androgenetic alopecia should report that their hair loss has been gradual, progressive, asymptomatic and not associated with any particular illness, stressor, or traumatic hairstyling practice. Any previous hair transplant surgeries should also be discussed (Table 1.2).

The patient's health status and surgical history should also be elicited. A comprehensive medical history should be documented. Discussion with a specialist or primary care physician may be advisable with any condition that can potentially affect the procedure. Although hair transplantation has low risk for complication, it is advisable that any patient over age 55 obtain medical clearance from their primary care physician. Their current medication list should also be carefully reviewed. The use of anticoagulant medication is a relative contraindication to the procedure. Hair transplantation can still be performed on anticoagulated patients. However, it can be more technically difficult. The lack of proper hemostasis may make graft planting more arduous, with increased oozing, decreased visibility, and more graft popping. The patient may consult with their primary care physician about discontinuing the medication prior to the procedure; however, risking a possible cardiovascular event for an elective procedure may be inadvisable. Even if the patient takes anticoagulants for prophylactic use, their primary care physician should approve of the medication's discontinuation.

Scalp Examination (Table 1.3)

A thorough scalp examination should help identify the type of alopecia, as well as determine if a patient

Table 1.1: History of previous transplant.
Suggested questions to obtain a detailed history during the consult
How long has the hair loss been present?
Is the hair loss sudden or gradual?
Is the hair loss localized or diffuse?
Is the hair loss associated with increased shedding?
Is there any associated itching, burning, tenderness, or oozing?
What aspect of the hair loss bothers you?
What are your expectations of the hair transplant?
What medications are you currently taking? Any anticoagulants used?
What medications are being taken to treat the hair loss?
Any previous surgeries, including hair transplants?
Do you currently smoke? If yes, how many packs per day?
Do you tend to develop keloids or hypertrophic scars?
Is there any current or previous use of traumatic hairstyling practice?

Table 1.2: Questions to elicit history.
Obtaining history of previous hair transplant
Which donor harvesting method was performed: strip excision or FUE?
Identify the recipient area. How many grafts were placed?
Was there adequate graft survival?
Were there any of complications? (i.e. widened scar)
Were there any aspects that they were dissatisfied with from the previous surgery?

(FUE: Follicular unit extraction).

Table 1.3: Scalp examination.
Determine Norwood-Hamilton or Ludwig classification
Note any presence of inflammation
Note any evidence of scarring hair loss
Evaluate previous donor scar
Evaluate donor density
Evaluate hair caliber
Note hair color
Evaluate scalp laxity

is an adequate candidate. In addition, the proposed recipient area can be outlined at that time. Moreover, the number of grafts that will be needed to restore the desired area can be approximated.

Evaluation of the Recipient Area

Clinically, androgenetic alopecia is an asymptomatic, patterned hair loss with miniaturized hairs and thinning in the affected areas. The hairs diminish from thick, pigmented terminal hairs into thin, fine vellus hairs. Male-patterned alopecia more commonly displays progressive frontotemporal hairline recession, as well as gradual thinning over the frontal and vertex scalp. If left untreated, smooth, bald scalp will develop in the affected areas. The most commonly used classification system to assess male-patterned hair loss is the Norwood-Hamilton scale (Fig. 1.4). In contrast, with female-patterned alopecia, the frontal hairline is preserved with gradual thinning and follicular miniaturization throughout the frontal scalp (Figs. 1.5A and B). This appearance is referred to as the "Christmas tree" pattern with a widened central part and a more "see-through" nature of the hair. Female-patterned hair loss rarely progresses to the point of developing smooth, bald areas. Female-patterned alopecia can be classified using the Ludwig

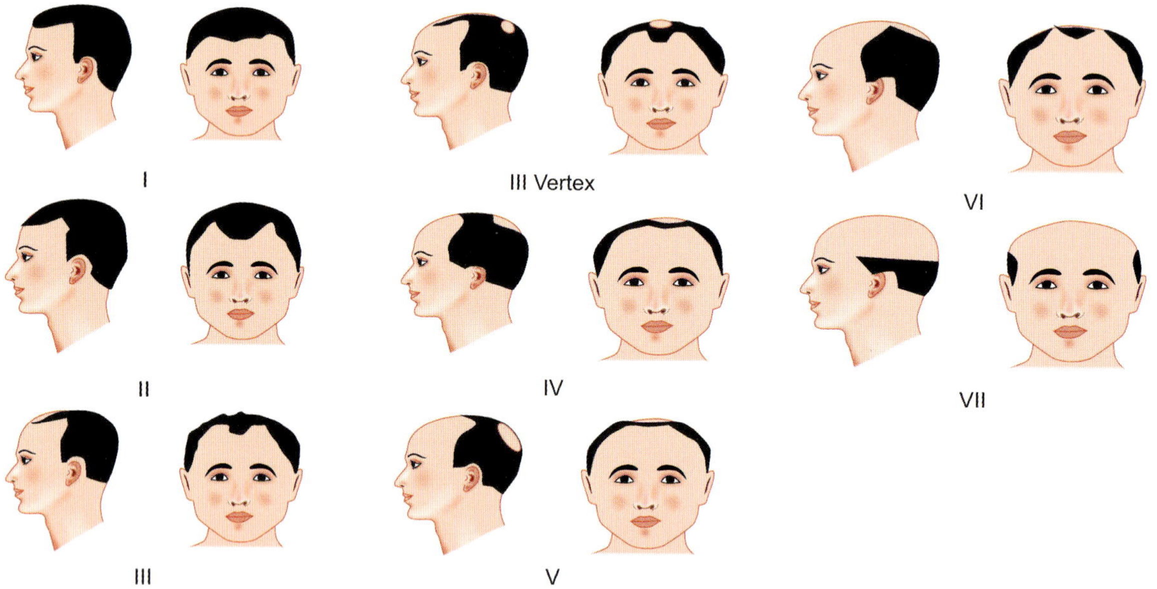

Fig. 1.4: Norwood-Hamilton classification scale for male-patterned hair loss.

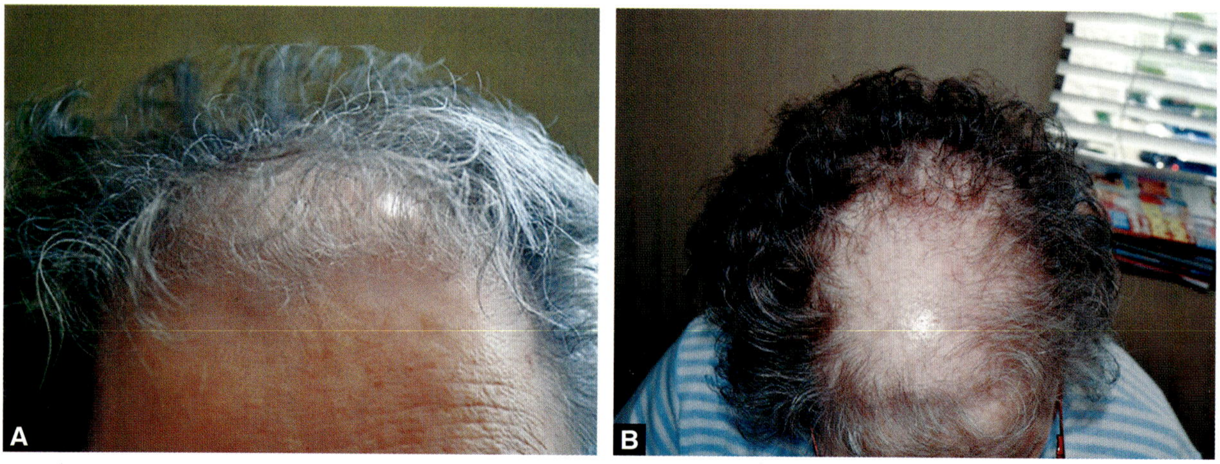

Figs. 1.5A and B: A woman with Ludwig type III female-patterned hair loss demonstrating preservation of the frontal hairline (A) with follicular miniaturization and increased central part width on the frontal scalp (B).

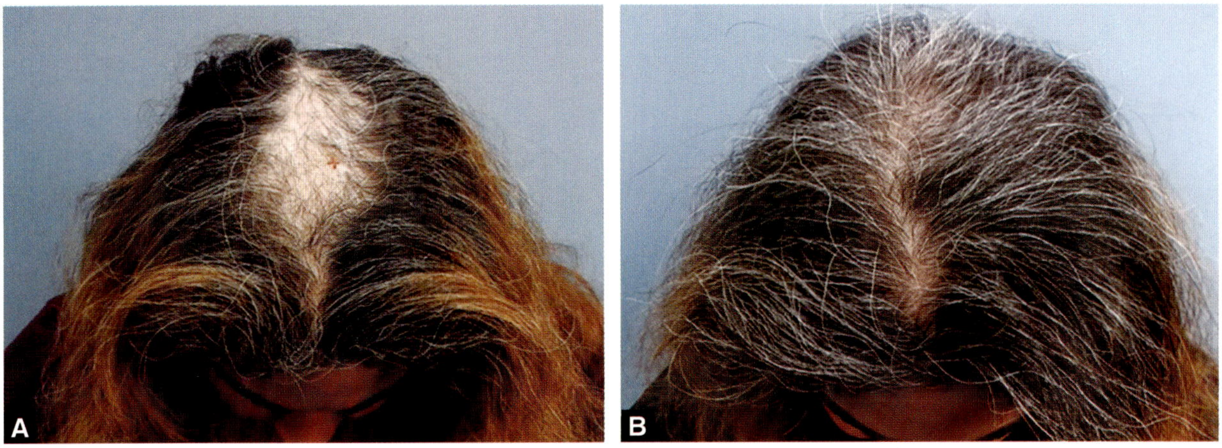

Figs. 1.6A and B: A 29-year-old woman seeking hair transplant consultation. (A) At initial visit with seemingly Ludwig type III female-patterned hair loss. Biopsy also confirmed Female pattern hair loss (FPHL). (B) However, within 5 months, her hair was restored to its previous state with minoxidil. Thus, she demonstrated telogen effluvium mimicking female-patterned hair loss.

scale. In females, there should be enough space to make incisions and place grafts without transecting the existing hair follicles. In addition, further workup, such as laboratory and histologic examination, may be warranted with any unusual presentation. Care should be given that patterned alopecia is distinguished from telogen effluvium or an inflammatory alopecia, such as lichen planopilaris or central centrifugal cicatricial alopecia (Figs. 1.6A and B).

Evaluation of the Donor Area (See Chapter 3)

The donor area refers to the designated zone from which the grafts will be harvested for transplantation. In order to successfully perform hair transplantation, adequate donor supply is necessary. Many factors dictate whether the donor area is suitable for graft extraction. The surgeon should be able to create enough grafts to provide the desired coverage in the recipient area. In addition, care should be given to avoid extracting grafts from an area where ongoing hair loss may eventually occur, as these grafts will not survive indefinitely. In addition, if strip excision is performed and ongoing hair loss occurs in the donor area, the linear scar may become visible.

Donor Area "Safe Zone"

The theory of donor dominance states that grafts harvested in areas unaffected by hair loss should maintain its same genetic destiny when transplanted into involved recipient areas, allowing them to grow indefinitely. Therefore, the grafts should be extracted from a donor area as immune to future hair loss as possible. In most individuals with androgenetic alopecia, there is a horse shoe shaped region along the occipital scalp that is less likely to be eventually affected by hair loss. This is considered the 'safe zone' and where most grafts are extracted for hair transplant (Fig. 1.7).

The 'safe zone' is defined as a 5-6 centimeter width, horseshoe-shaped band stretching across the occipital scalp, extending into the temporal scalp. It can be more precisely approximated by drawing a horizontal line in between the superior aspects of the ear helices to create the superior border. The occipital notches or nuchal ridges defines the inferior border. Extending the strip below this line seems to increase the risk for a widened scar. The lateral borders of the safe zone should extend no further than the temporal scalp above the superior ear helices. It is advisable to harvest approximately 2 cm from the superior and inferior borders, as the thinning may eventually progress to expose the linear scar.

Care should be taken to correctly identify the unaffected area in women with diffuse androgenetic alopecia. With "patterned" alopecia in females, the central part width should be widened in the frontal scalp compared to the occipital scalp. With diffuse alopecia, the occipital scalp may appear as thinned and the "see-through" nature may be just as apparent. This is a relative contraindication for graft harvesting in the typical "safe zone" in these individuals, as the grafts will have already begun to miniaturize and may not survive indefinitely. It is possible to estimate the extent and rate of hairloss in individuals with androgenetic alopecia. For example, a 60-year-old

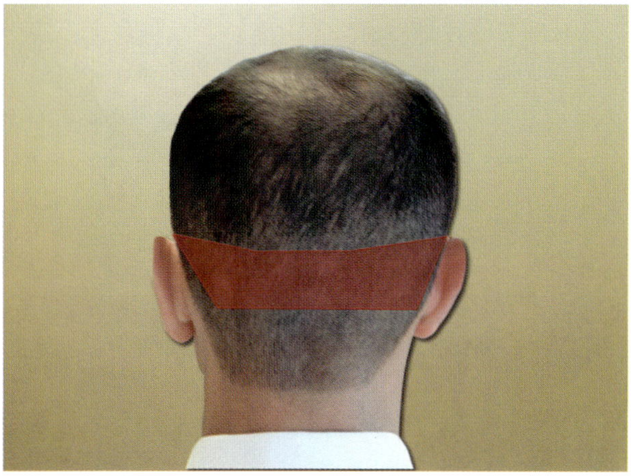

Fig. 1.7: Safe donor area

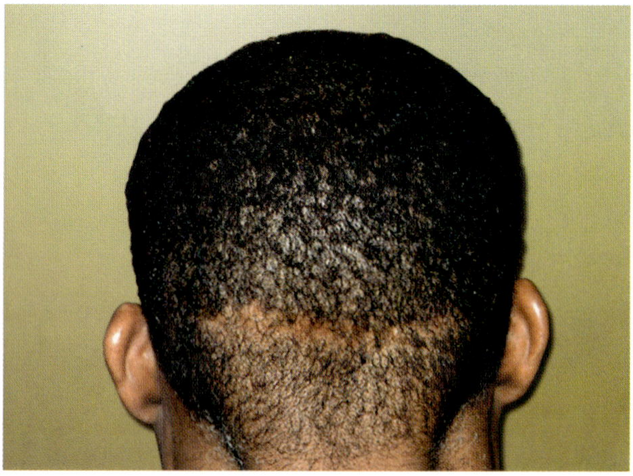

Fig. 1.8: Demonstrating a visibly, widened scar on an African-American man that wears a very short hairstyle.

man with a slow, progression to a Norwood III level alopecia is unlikely to develop severe, Norwoood VI alopecia. Likewise, it can be assumed that a young, 22-year-old man with Norwood III hairloss is at high-risk to eventually develop end stage Norwood VII alopecia. These individuals would not be good candidates for strip excision because the linear scar may become visible. In addition, the transplanted grafts may not survive indefinitely.

Examination of Previous Donor Area

Many patients have undergone previous hair transplant surgeries. If strip excision was performed previously, the prior scar(s) should be examined. Any complication should be noted, including wound dehiscence, infection, widened scar or keloid formation (Fig. 1.8). Moreover, the donor area should be evaluated for adequate donor supply and laxity surrounding the previous scar. The subsequent surgery may include the area containing the previous scar. Follicles with surrounding fibrosis may not achieve adequate survival. If follicular unit extraction (FUE) was previously performed, the donor area should be examined for the possible presence of hypopigmented macular scarring. Also it is possible to overharvest with FUE, creating a thinned, moth-eaten appearance to the donor area.

Donor Density

Density is defined by the number of follicular units per square centimeter as opposed to hairs per square centimeter. There are numerous methods and devices to approximate the donor density. An easy method is to count the number of follicular units in a 0.25 square centimeter area and multiply by four, acknowledging that the density is not uniform throughout the entire donor area. The ideal candidate has a donor density of at least 70-90 follicular units per square centimeter. Densities of less than 40 follicular units per square centimeter have poor donor supply.

Caliber

The hair caliber is an important characteristic to assess as well. The hair caliber affects the perceived density of the final cosmetic outcome. Any hair follicle greater than 70 microns is considered a thick caliber hair. Thick, kinky-curly hairs provide greater coverage than fine, straight hairs. An individual with thin, straight hair may need as much twice as many transplanted grafts to create the same perceived density (Figs. 1.9A and B). Conversely, individuals with thick-curly hair with limited donor areas are considered fortunate as they will not need as many grafts to provide adequate coverage of the desired recipient area. This concept can be useful in patients with central centrifugal cicatricial alopecia (CCCA) for example. To create an increased perceived density in individuals with thin, wispy hair, a greater number of larger 3-4 follicular unit grafts can be transplanted in the recipient area. Moreover, women with kinky-curly hair should be discouraged to use chemical relaxers on the hair postoperatively as this will significantly reduce the perceived density.

Scalp Elasticity

Scalp elasticity is also a major determinant of potential donor supply with the strip excision method. The main risk factor for widened, hypertrophic scarring

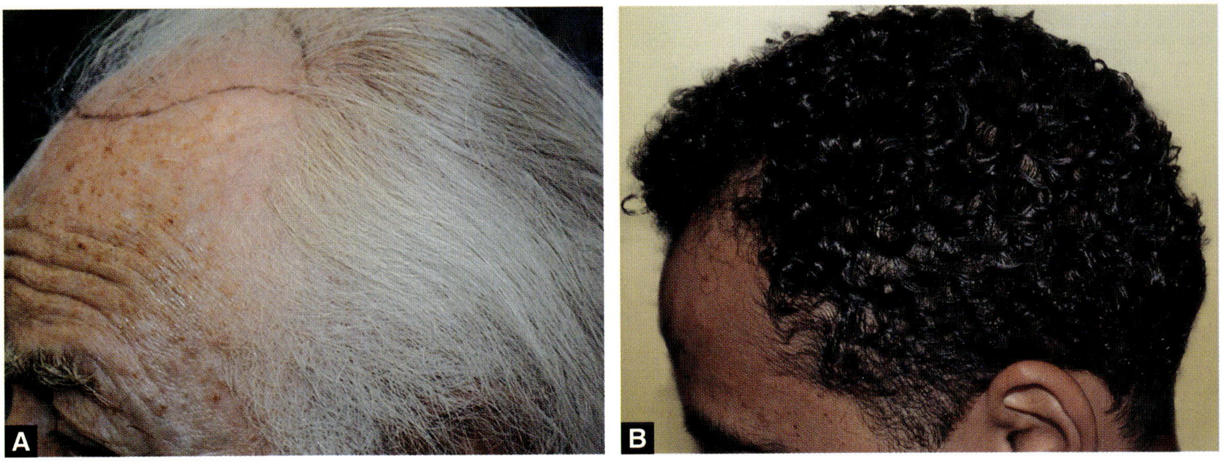

Figs. 1.9A and B: (A) Demonstrating fine, wispy gray hair on light colored scalp. (B) Thick, curly black hair on darker scalp.

Table 1.4: Using the Mayer-Paul's formula to determine the maximum strip width that can be extracted.

Scalp elasticity (%)	*Maximum strip width (cm)*
10	1
15	1.5
20	2
25	2.5

is wound tension. With greater scalp laxity, a wider strip maybe safely extracted, increasing the number of harvested grafts. Maintaining a maximum strip width of less than 1 cm decreases the risk of widened scars. However, if the scalp is tight or a larger session with a strip greater than 1 cm width is desired, then properly assessing the scalp elasticity is warranted. The Mayer-Pauls formula is a helpful measurement of scalp elasticity and is used to determine the maximum donor width. The surgeon places their thumb and index finger 5 cm apart and compresses the scalp skin together. The percentage change from the original distance to the compressed distance is measured (D) (Table 1.4).

$$\% \text{ Scalp elasticity} = (50 \text{ mm} - D) / 50 \text{ mm} \times 100$$

Hair Color

Hair color of the donor area can affect graft slivering as well as the final cosmetic outcome. With regards to slivering, it can be more difficult to readily identify the entire subcutaneous course of gray hairs, especially if curly, leading to increased transaction rates. This may be avoided by staining the follicles with Gentian violet.

Even with adequate perceived density in the recipient area, individuals with very dark hair and a very light colored scalp may appear to have a more see-through effect or decreased density. The dark hairs can highlight the light colored scalp, causing it to become more perceptible. In addition, any complication in the recipient area such as pitting, a too straight hairline, or textural change maybe noticeable. Therefore, patients with very light scalps should be advised to dye their hair lighter. Conversely, individuals with darker scalps should keep their hair darker. Ideally, the more the hair color approximates the scalp color, a see-through nature in the recipient area can be avoided.

Key Concepts for the Donor Area

- An ideal hair transplant candidate has adequate donor supply to cover the desired recipient area
- If present, the previous donor scar should be examined
- Both donor density and hair caliber determine the final perceived density
- Scalp elasticity should be evaluated if a strip excision is being performed
- Hair color should be lighter on fair skin and darker on dark skin.

Details to review with the patient: The preoperative course and instructions should be reviewed with the patient (Table 1.5). If the patient chooses to undergo the follicular unit extraction procedure, they should be counseled preoperatively about trimming the hairs. Typically, a large 5–6 cm wide band will need to be trimmed for donor harvesting. However, depending on the original length, it may

Table 1.5: Preoperative course.
Review the consent
Photographs are taken
Discontinue aspirin
Discontinue minoxidil one week prior to the procedure
Hair trimmed as needed

Table 1.7: Postoperative course.
Dressing removed the next day
Recipient area shampooed gently
Oral prednisone 40 mg x 3 days PRN to reduce edema
Vicodin x 7 days
Postoperative antibiotics as needed
Sutures or staples removed in 7 days if strip excision performed
Grafts may shed 2–3 weeks postoperatively
Use of minoxidil and/or low level light stimulation to potentially improve growth and reduce risk of postoperative telogen effluvium as needed
Restart medications to control ongoing hair loss
Full cosmetic effect can be expected 9–18 months later

take several weeks to grow the hair back. Therefore, patients may choose to allow the whole head to be shaved or simply tapered low in the back to mask the area. Alternatively, they may choose to grow the hair several centimeters long to mask the shaved area.

The details of the procedure should also be discussed with the patient. They should be informed that hair transplantation is an outpatient procedure, performed under local anesthesia by the surgeon and their team of technicians. The discussion should include the type of donor harvesting method used, how the grafts are created and inserted, and the approximate duration of the procedure. All risks and potential complications should also be explained (Table 1.6).

Graft survival depends on the technical aspects of the surgery, as well as the postoperative care. The grafts should be protected from trauma and the adherent scabs should not be picked. Therefore, it is important to thoroughly review the postoperative care and expected course (Table 1.7).

In summary, the consult and preoperative evaluation are determining factors in the success of hair transplant. The final outcome should appear natural and is determined by the donor supply, hair caliber, and control of the ongoing hair loss (Table 1.8).

Table 1.6: Potential risks and complications from hair transplant.
Folliculitis
Cysts
Wound dehiscence
Infection
Neuropathic pain from strip excision
Ischemic necrosis in the recipient area—risk increased with dense packing and in smokers
Unnatural appearance
Poor graft survival

Table 1.8: Key concepts.
Transplant should appear natural
The grafts survive due to the theory of donor dominance
Two methods of harvesting: strip excision vs FUE
Strip excision causes a visible, linear scar
With FUE, a large area is shaved with the risk for diffuse, hypopigmented macular scars
The donor supply is limited
The perceived density is a function of both the density of grafts placed and hair caliber
The net cosmetic outcome is the number of grafts placed with hair transplant minus ongoing hair loss

(FUE: Follicular unit extraction).

Finally, if the patient decides to schedule the procedure, a packet with detailed pre- and post-operative instructions, prescriptions for postoperative medications, and a detailed consent form is sent. Patients are encouraged to call with any concerns prior to the procedure.

BIBLIOGRAPHY

1. Avram MR, Keene SA, Dowling Stough & Nicole E Rogers, et al. Hair restoration. Dermatology. 2012; 2:2535-45.
2. Avram MR, Rogers NE. The consult, preoperative period, instrumentation and anesthesia setup, and postoperative period. In: Hair Transplantation. Cambridge University Press; 2010.
3. Fisher J. Hair restoration. Plast Surg. 2013;2: 494-506.
4. Griffin TD. Hair transplantation. J Am Acad Dermatol. 2011;66:170-71.
5. Jimenez F. The Donor Area. Hair Transplantation. New York: Cambridge University Press. 2010; pp.15–21
6. Konior RJ. Hair restoration: medical and surgical techniques. Cummings Otolaryngol. 2014;1:371-90.

CHAPTER

2

Preoperative and Postoperative Instructions for Hair Transplant Surgery

Shannon Watkins, Marc R Avram

PREOPERATIVE WORKUP

Before performing a hair transplant surgery in healthy patients under the age of 55 years old, no medical clearance is typically required. For those patients 55 years or older, we require medical clearance from a primary doctor as well as an electrocardiogram (EKG). Medical clearance is also required for younger patients with pre-existing medical conditions such as diabetes and/or known cardiac issues. For females of childbearing age, we also require a beta-human chorionic gonadotropin (β-HCG) pregnancy test prior to surgery to confirm the patients is not pregnant, as many medications used during the procedure are not approved for pregnancy. *See* Table 2.1 for a summary of our preoperative workup.

Once the patient decides to go forward with the surgery, we have them fill out a health questionnaire, *see* Table 2.2 for a sample health questionnaire. On the day of the surgery, we have them fill out an additional health questionnaire asking about details pertinent to their surgery such as if they have taken their preoperative antibiotics (if indicated), had any sedatives in the past day (which may influence the preoperative sedatives we administer), or consumed any alcohol or used Rogaine in the past 24 hours (which may increase their intraoperative bleeding risk). *See* Table 2.3 for the day of surgery health questionnaire.

Table 2.1: Preoperative workup for hair transplant surgery.

Medical clearance from primary doctor for all patients 55 years and older (male and female)
Medical clearance from primary doctor for patients younger than 55 years old with pre-existing medical conditions such as but not limited to diabetes and/or known cardiac conditions
Pregnancy test performed on all females of childbearing age

We also discuss possible complications with patients and have them sign a consent form prior to the day of their surgery. *See* Table 2.4 for a list of complications from hair transplant surgery. *See* Table 2.5 for a list of the key points a hair transplant surgery consent form should address.

ANTICOAGULANTS

Patients on anticoagulants such as aspirin, warfarin, vitamin E, rivaroxaban, dabigatran, apixaban are asked to speak with their primary doctor and/or cardiologist to see if the anticoagulants can safely be discontinued prior to surgery. For many patients, these medications are medically necessary and cannot be discontinued. If this is the case, the hair transplant surgery is not performed due to increased risk of bleeding complications. For those patients who are medically able to discontinue their anticoagulant medications, we ask them to discontinue them 10 days prior to the hair transplant procedure.

Alcohol is also an anticoagulant, so we ask patient to refrain from alcohol for 24 hours prior to and 1–3 days after the procedure.

Table 2.2: Sample health questionnaire for hair transplant surgery—completed prior to day of surgery.

Sample health questionnaire—done prior to day of surgery	*Yes*	*No*	*N/A*
Are you allergic to any drugs or medications? If so please list the drugs and the reactions:			
Have you ever had a severe allergic reaction to anything? If so please list what the substance and the reaction were:			
Have you ever had any of the following: (1) heart disease, (2) high blood pressure, (3) hepatitis, and (4) ulcer disease?			
Do you have any other chronic health conditions? If so, please list them:			
Have you had a blood transfusion in the last 10 years?			
In the past 6 months have you taken any of the following: 1. Steroids 2. Birth control pills 3. Antibiotics 4. Anticoagulants 5. Thyroid medications 6. Heart medication 7. Aspirin/Advil 8. Tranquilizers/antidepressants 9. Narcotics/pain medications 10. Diabetic medication 11. Blood pressure medication 12. Vitamins If yes, then which ones:			
Are you being treated for any medical problems at this time? Do you have a history of any of the following: 1. Cardiac problems (high blood pressure, heart attack, heart valve problems, palpitations/irregular heart beat, heart disease, chest pain) 2. Diabetes 3. Thyroid problems 4. Liver and/or kidney problems 5. Infections (herpes, hepatitis, impetigo) 6. Convulsions or epilepsy 7. Asthma 8. Bleeding tendencies Are your pregnant? Date of last menstrual period ______________ Do you have a history of any other medical problems? If so please list below:			
Do you have any prior hospitalizations and/or surgeries? If so please list below:			
Do you smoke? If so how much?			
Do you drink alcohol? If so how much?			
Have you ever experienced an unusual reaction to anesthesia? If so, what?			
Is there anything else we should be aware of not listed in this history? If so what?			

PROPHYLACTIC ANTIBIOTICS

Antibiotic prophylaxis is not typically indicated for hair transplant surgery, as it is considered a clean procedure. Some hair transplant surgeons, however, administer prophylactic antibiotics to patients at a higher risk of infection such as immunocompromised patients and patients with diabetes. Many surgeons also give prophylactic antibiotics for patients at increased risk of prosthetic joint infections such as those in the first 2 years following a joint replacement, or those with a history of previous prosthetic joint infections. Patients who are at an increased risk of endocarditis may also receive prophylactic antibiotics for conditions such as a prosthetic cardiac valve, a history of previous infective endocarditis, certain congenital heart diseases, and cardiac transplant patients who develop a cardiac valvulopathy. Again, the surgery is only performed if the patient gets medical clearance from his/her primary doctor.[1] *See* Table 2.6 for a list of conditions for which pre-operative antibiotics can be considered for hair transplant surgery.

Table 2.3: Sample health questionnaire—day of surgery.

Sample health questionnaire—day of surgery	*Yes*	*No*	*N/A*
Have you taken your antibiotic (if indicated)?			
Have you consumed any alcohol in the past 24 hours?			
Have you consumed vitamin E, aspirin, or any anticoagulants in the past 10 days?			
Have you taken any prescription sedatives or anxiolytic agents in the past 24 hours?			
Do you use, or have you ever used Rogaine?			
Did you use Rogaine in the past 24 hours?			
Have you read the instruction sheet?			
Are you allergic to any drugs or medications? If so please list the drug and the reaction:			
Have you ever had a severe allergic Reaction to anything? If so please list the substance and the reaction:			
Have you ever had any of the following: (1) heart disease, (2) high blood pressure, (3) hepatitis, and (4) ulcer disease?			
Do you have any other chronic health conditions? If so, please list them:			
Have you had a blood transfusion in the last 10 years?			
Have you had a temperature to 100.4°F or higher in the past week? If so, when was the last fever?			
Have you had any recent changes in your health, or any active medical conditions in the past week?			
Did you eat breakfast this morning?			

Table 2.4: List of complications from hair transplant surgery. Patient should sign a consent form, stating he/she has read and understands all the possible complications listed below.

More common complications	*Rare complications (partial list only)*
Nausea and vomiting from pain medication	Keloid formation in donor area
Bleeding (<5%)	Complete failure of growth of transplanted hair
Infection (<1%)	Persistent scalp pain
Excessive swelling/bruising	Total loss of donor hair
Temporary headache	Permanent numbness of scalp
Temporary numbness of scalp	Noticeable scarring of donor area
Scarring around grafts	Allergic reaction or medication—related problems
Allergic reactions to medications (<1%)	Other unforeseen medical emergencies may arise
Fainting (<1%)	
Small in grown hair, causing a cyst (<10%)	
Temporary or permanent loss of existing hair in transplanted region of scalp	

When indicated, prophylactic antibiotics should be taken 30–60 minutes prior to the procedure. For nonpenicillin allergic patients, the typical regimen is cephalexin 2 g or dicloxacillin 2 g orally. In patients with a penicillin allergy, clindamycin 600 mg, azithromycin 500 mg, or clarithromycin 500 mg can be given orally. If there is an increased risk of methicillin-resistant *Staphylococcus aureus* (MRSA) in the community, a physician can consider one tablet of Bactrim Double Strength and Penicillin-VK 500 mg or Clindamycin 600 mg orally prior to the procedure.[1] *See* Table 2.7 for a summary of preoperative antibiotic regimens recommended for skin surgery.

PREOPERATIVE INSTRUCTIONS FOR HAIR TRANSPLANT SURGERY

Patients who are having local anesthesia for their hair transplant surgery are advised to eat a good meal prior to their procedure. Patients are advised to avoid alcoholic beverages for 24 hours prior to and for 1–3 days after the procedure due to increased bleeding risk. They are also instructed to discontinue Rogaine

Table 2.5: Key points a hair transplant surgery consent form should address.
Consent for the surgery and any services that become necessary during the procedure.
Statement that patient is aware that more than one hair transplant procedure may be necessary. Physician should estimate that (X) number of procedures is estimated to be necessary for satisfactory results.
Statement that there is no guarantee of good growth or good cosmetic results, as there will likely be ongoing hair loss, and variables such as donor hair availability and donor hair quality will affect the result.
Statement that patient has read and understands: (1) complications and (2) pre- and post-operative instructions.
Statement that patients understands the procedure and reasonable results and that they will not have a full head of hair after the procedure.
Statement that there will be scarring associated with the procedure that is typically not visible but that will be visible if the hair is shaved.
Statement that patient is aware that complications may occur (patient is given a list of possible complications, *see* Table 2.4 for a list of complications from hair transplant surgery).
Statement that patient consents to administration of local anesthesia or IV solutions if it is necessary.
Statement that patient authorizes the performance of the hair transplant surgery by the stated MD and his/her hair transplant assistants
Statement that patient has been well informed and understands cosmetic surgery results cannot be guaranteed.
Statement that the pros/cons/alternatives to the hair transplant surgery including doing nothing at all, wearing a hairpiece or wig, using medications, or a combination of the above. These pros/cons/alternatives have been discussed.
Statement that future hair loss will likely occur and that it may affect the appearance of transplanted hair. Though transplanted hairs are usually long-lasting in some cases, they have been noted to fall out after 1–10 years. A small percentage of men (<10%) do loose majority of the donor hair, which can affect final results and make the donor scar visible.
Statement that patient has been advised that Rogaine and/or Propecia will help hold onto existing hair and regrow hair, and if patient does not choose to use medications, it will affect the perceived density and appearance of hair after transplant surgery.
Statement that this consent was signed and read without the influence of medications that may cause drowsiness.
Statement that the procedure and form has been fully explained to patient, it is understood, and that patient understands all contents of the consent form.

Table 2.6: Patients to consider preoperative antibiotics for hair transplant surgery.
Immunocompromised patients
Patients with diabetes
Patients with a history of a joint replacement in the past 2 years
Patients with a history of a previous joint infection
Patients at an increased risk for endocarditis
Patients with certain congenital heart disease
Cardiac transplant patients with a cardiac valvulopathy

for 7 days prior and 3 days after the surgery due to potential vasodilatory properties of Rogaine leading to increased bleeding risk. They are also advised to discontinue any anticoagulants 10 days prior to their procedure, as long as this has been approved by their primary doctor. Propecia may be continued during the surgery.

We also ask patients to inform us if they have a temperature over 100.4°F or any other active medical conditions that arise prior to their surgery day.

Table 2.7: Preoperative antibiotic regimens for skin surgery.

	Nonpenicillin allergic	*Penicillin allergic*
Community with low MRSA prevalence	Cephalexin 2 g or Dicloxacillin 2 g	Clindamycin 600 mg or Azithromycin 500 mg or Clarithromycin 500 mg
Community with high MRSA prevalence	Bactrim DS PO and Penicillin-VK 500 mg	Clindamycin 600 mg

(MRSA: Methicillin-resistant *Staphylococcus aureus*; DS: Double strength).

See Table 2.8 for a summary of preoperative instructions given to patients prior to their procedure.

POSTOPERATIVE INSTRUCTIONS FOR HAIR TRANSPLANT SURGERY

Patients leave the office with a bandage in place. We recommend they keep the bandage in place until the following day. Patients who have taken valium

Table 2.8: Hair replacement surgery preoperative instructions.
Discontinue vitamin E, Coumadin, aspirin, and any other anticoagulants (as long as okay with your primary doctor or the prescribing physician) 10 days prior to the procedure. If you are taking the medication for a medical condition, always consult with the prescribing physician prior to discontinuing a medication.
Do not consume alcoholic beverages for 24 hours prior to the procedure, and for 1–3 days after the procedure, due to increased bleeding risk.
Discontinue Rogaine 7 days prior to the procedure, and wait 3 days after the procedure to resume Rogaine use. This should not result in any hair loss.
Propecia may be continued.
Women of childbearing age must have a negative pregnancy test (β-HCG) prior to the surgery.
Men and women 55 years and over must have medical clearance from their primary medical doctor (PMD), including an ECG.
Men and women under the age of 55 years old, with any active medical issues, must also have clearance from their primary doctor.
Please advise us if you have a temperature of 100.4°F or higher, or any other active medical conditions that may arise in the week prior to your surgery.
If prescribed an antibiotic, please take it 30–60 minutes prior to your surgery.
Please eat a meal prior to coming to the office, if you are doing the procedure under local anesthesia.
If you are having the procedure done under IV sedation, DO NOT have food or drink after midnight the night before the procedure.
Please wear a button down shirt to the surgery, so nothing will interfere with your bandage.

(ECG: Electrocardiography; IV: Intravenous; β-HCG: Beta-human chorionic gonadotropin).

Table 2.9: Postoperative medications given for hair transplant surgery.
Tylenol with Codeine #3 (300 mg Tylenol/30 mg Codeine) Sig: 1 tablet every 4–6 hours PRN pain Disp: 6 tablets
Prednisone 40 mg tablet* Sig: 1 tablet PO night of procedure, then QAM x 2 days Disp: 3 tablets

*Only given for procedure of the frontal scalp to avoid swelling of the forehead/face.

or another sedative agent are instructed not to drive or take public transportation. They should be accompanied home by a responsible adult.

We instruct patients to shower daily starting the day after their surgery, and to let water run gently over their scalp. It is emphasized that they should not pick at the scabs, which should resolve in the following 1-2 weeks after hair transplant surgery as picking at the scabs could lead to loss of the transplanted hair.

Patients are advised to avoid heavy lifting and strenuous exercise for at least 4 days, ideally 7 days after their surgery. For the first 48 hours, we recommend they avoid leaning over to tie shoes/pick up objects on the floor due to increased bleeding risk. We also advise them to avoid alcoholic beverages for 24 hours postoperative to minimize the bleeding risk.

We prescribe them Tylenol #3 which they can take every 4-6 hours as needed for pain with food to minimize nausea. They can also take extra strength Tylenol as indicated on the package label if the pain is not very severe. For patients who have the hair transplant procedure performed on their frontal scalp, we also prescribe prednisone 40 mg tablets, once daily for 3 days to minimize postoperative edema and swelling of the forehead and face. They are instructed to take the first tablet the afternoon or evening of the surgery and the subsequent tablets in the morning for the next 2 days. Patients are instructed that if they do get some forehead and facial edema, this is routine and will self-resolve in the next few days. Prednisone is not routinely given for hair transplant surgeries of areas other than the frontal scalp, as forehead and facial edema does not seem to be common after surgeries in these locations. *See* Table 2.9 for a list of postoperative medications given for hair transplant surgery.

If bleeding occurs, we instruct them to apply firm steady pressure through the bandage for 15 minutes. If bleeding still persists, this is repeated for 15 more minutes. If bleeding still persists, we instruct them to remove the bandage and locate exact bleeding point

Table 2.10: Postoperative instructions for hair transplant surgery.
Please arrange transportation from the office. You cannot drive or take public transportation by yourself, as you will most likely have taken a sedative. Please have a friend or relative pick you up from the office after the surgery. If you are unable to have someone pick you up, please notify the office in advance.
Eat something after leaving the office.
Take the prescribed Tylenol #3 with food to avoid nausea. Do not wait until you have pain.
Avoid heavy lifting and strenuous exercise for at least 4 days after the surgery, ideally for 7 days after surgery. Do not lean over to tie your shoes, or pick up objects from the floor for the first 48 hours, as this may provoke bleeding.
Do not drink alcohol for 24 hours prior to and 1–3 days after the hair transplant procedure. Avoid all nonprescribed chemical substances for 4 days after surgery.
Get a good night sleep. Sleep with one or two pillows to elevate your head if possible.
If bleeding occurs, apply firm pressure through the bandage for 15 minutes. If bleeding still persists, hold firm pressure again for another 15 minutes. If there is still bleeding, remove the bandage and locate the exact point of bleeding, and apply direct pressure to this area for 15 minutes. The pressure should be firm and steady. If bleeding has not stopped at this point, please call the office, or if you are out of town go to the nearest emergency room.
The day after the surgery, remove the dressing (it should come off easily since there is no adhesive). There will be small scabs present around the transplanted hairs, DO NOT PICK THE SCABS OFF, as this can damage transplanted follicles. Take a shower. Allow the water to gently run over the transplanted hair, but do not rub or scratch the area. Do not shampoo the transplanted region, you may shampoo the side and back of the scalp. You may gently shampoo the transplanted region 2 days after the surgery if you feel comfortable.
Apply Bacitracin or Aquaphor ointment once to twice daily to the donor region (the back of the scalp) for 1 week, or until the stables or sutures are removed. Scabs will form over the transplant sites and solidify over the first few days, again DO NOT SCRATCH OR PICK THESE OFF, doing so can damage the transplanted hairs. They will fall off naturally within 1–2 weeks.
If you are prescribed prednisone to minimize postoperative edema (swelling) of the forehead and eyes, take the first prednisone tablet the afternoon/night of the surgery. Then take one prednisone tablet each morning for the next 2 days. You will take prednisone for 3 days total. This should minimize swelling in the forehead area. If swelling does occur, this is not serious and it will resolve on its own over a few days.
Return to the office 7–10 days after the surgery to remove surgical staples or sutures. Full physical activities can be resumed after removal of the staples.
The transplanted hairs will begin to grow in 6–9 months after the procedure. The full results of the hair transplant will be seen 10–14 months after the procedure. You should schedule a follow-up appointment during this period.
Please destroy or return to the office any unused medications (Tylenol #3, prednisone, antibiotics), they are for your use only.
Please call us at the office in case of an emergency.

and apply direct pressure for 15 minutes. If this does not stop bleeding, we recommend they contact our office or go to the nearest emergency room.

POSTOPERATIVE WOUND CARE

We recommend that the day after the surgery, patients remove the bandage and shower. They are instructed to let water run gently over the transplanted area. They may gently shampoo the back and side of the scalp, but are instructed to avoid the transplanted area on the first day after surgery. On postoperative day 2, the patient may gently shampoo recipient area if they wish. They are advised to avoid picking off scabs in the recipient area, as this may damage the transplanted hair follicles. Patients are also instructed to apply Aquaphor or Bacitracin ointment twice daily to the donor area on the posterior scalp for 7 days until the sutures or staples are removed.

We advise patients that the transplanted hair will grow in 6–9 months after procedure. Full results are seen 10–14 months after the procedure. We recommend they schedule a follow-up appointment with us about 1 year after their procedure. *See* Table 2.10 for a summary of postoperative instructions given to patients after hair transplant surgery.

REFERENCE

1. Wright TI, Baddour LM, Berbari EF, et al. Antibiotic prophylaxis in dermatologic surgery: advisory statement 2008. J Am Acad Dermatol. 2008;59(3):464-73.

CHAPTER

3

Donor Harvesting in Hair Transplantation

Shannon Watkins

The quantity of donor hair is the limiting factor in hair transplantation surgery. This will likely remain true until hair can be cloned. Therefore, efficiency in donor harvesting is essential to avoid wasting a limited donor supply.

Hair transplantation is based on the concept of donor dominance suggested by Orentreich in 1959, which is the concept that hair retains the genetic makeup of the donor site, even after being transplanted.[1,2] This is important because in male- and female pattern hair loss, hair tends to be lost primarily from the top of the scalp (frontal, parietal, and vertex scalp) and retained in the posterior scalp. Donor dominance allows for hairs to be taken from the posterior scalp, where hairs will often remain for the duration of a patient's life, and placed on the top of scalp where they will last for many years. If a patient's posterior scalp hair is genetically determined to thin over time, it will thin whether it is in the posterior scalp or transplanted to the frontal scalp.[3]

There are many important aspects of donor harvesting in hair transplantation surgery. We discuss the various methods and techniques of donor harvesting in following sections.

A BRIEF HISTORY OF DONOR HARVESTING

From the 1960s to the mid-1990s, 3–4 mm punch biopsies were the standard method utilized to harvest hairs for transplantation. This technique was inefficient and labor intensive and created extensive scarring.[4] In the 1990s, elliptical donor strip harvesting became the standard method for harvesting hair from the posterior scalp and is still a popular method of donor harvesting today.[4,5] Starting in the early 2000s, follicular unit extraction (FUE) gained popularity as a method of harvesting hairs in their natural groupings of one to three hairs for use in hair transplantation. Follicular unit extraction is minimally invasive and offers the advantage of avoiding a linear scar on the posterior scalp, which is inevitable with elliptical donor harvesting. We will review in further detail elliptical donor strip harvesting and FUE, as these are the primary methods used for donor harvesting today.

IDEAL LOCATION FOR DONOR HARVESTING

One of the most important factors in hair transplantation is harvesting donor hair from a site that will not fall prey to ongoing hair loss. A safe donor area is one that is expected to be covered with hair for the lifetime of an individual, and therefore provide lasting coverage when transplanted.[2]

The "safe" donor area has three significant boundaries. The anterior boundary is thought to be vertically superior to the external acoustic meatus (Fig. 3.1A). The superior boundary is located 1–2 cm above the horizontal plane connecting the upper border of the helical rims. The inferior border is the occipital protuberance; as the inferior margin of the hairline may move upward with the progression of male and female hair loss (Fig. 3.1B).[2,3,6,7] One article by Park et al. suggests that the location of the parietal whorl may also be used to estimate the eventual progression of vertex alopecia. Based on a survey of 1,008 Korean males, they estimate that alopecia mostly progresses within 6 cm of the parietal whorl on the

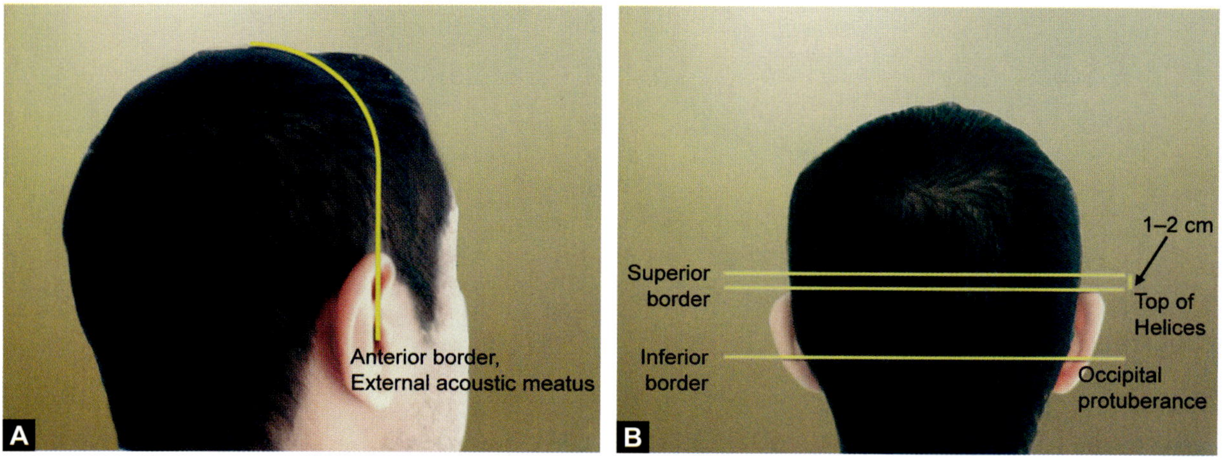

Figs. 3.1A and B: (A) Safe donor area, anterior border. Determined by line drawn vertically from external acoustic meatus. (B) Safe donor area, superior and inferior border. Inferior border determined by location of the occipital protuberance. Superior border is 1–2 cm above a horizontal line drawn from the top of the ear helices.

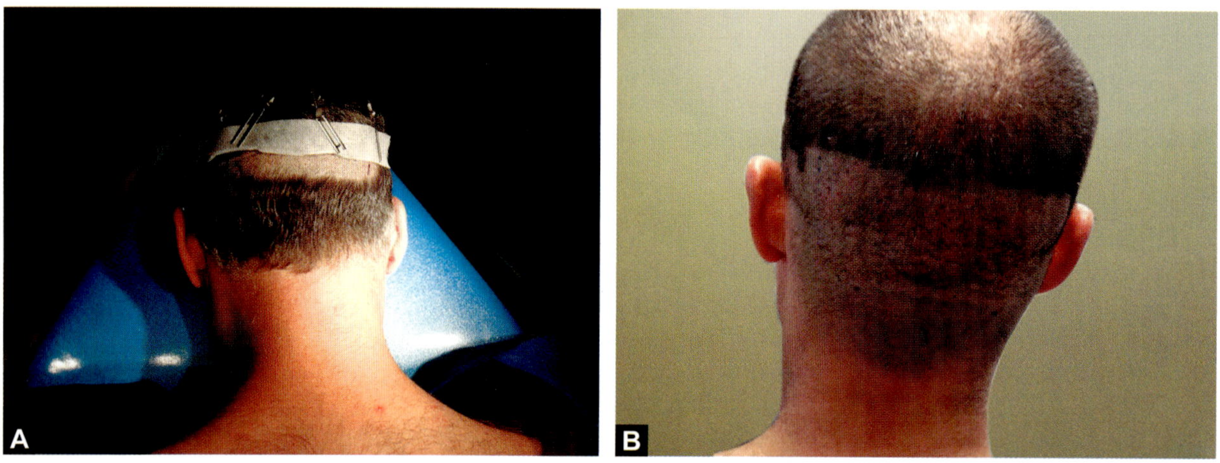

Figs. 3.2A and B: (A) Donor site for strip harvesting. (A) Donor site for follicular unit extraction (FUE) harvesting. Note the larger shaved area necessary for FUE harvesting.

occipital side. Therefore, the safe zone for donor harvesting may vary based on the location of a patient's parietal whorl. This 6 cm measurement may vary in Caucasians and other races, given their different facial structure; so before this becomes a clinical tool, further studies are needed.[2]

PREPARATION FOR DONOR HARVESTING

For patients undergoing elliptical donor strip harvesting, we recommend they wear their hair at least 2–3 cm long on the posterior scalp so that their hair will camouflage the sutures or staples placed during the procedure. The donor region is trimmed 2–3 mm long with a moustache trimmer (Fig. 3.2A).

For patients undergoing FUE, we encourage them to shave the hair on their posterior scalp short. The day of the procedure, a mustache trimmer is used to trim a larger donor area on the posterior scalp to a length of 1 mm (Fig. 3.2B). This area is typically too large to be concealed by longer hairs as with the elliptical donor strip harvesting. A few days after the procedure, once surgical sites have healed we instruct them to visit their barber to fade or blend the edges.

We harvest donor hair while patients are in a prone position. This allows for better visibility and stability. It also decreases the incidence of vasovagal episodes while harvesting.[3]

ANESTHESIA FOR DONOR HARVESTING

Briefly, the donor area is anesthetized with 1% lidocaine with epinephrine 1:100,000. Saline (10–30 mL) is then added for increased turgor to assist with anesthesia, hemostasis, and reduce hair follicle transection during harvesting. Anesthesia and instrumentation will be discussed in more detail in Chapter 5.[3]

ELLIPTICAL DONOR STRIP HARVESTING

In elliptical donor strip harvesting, a scalpel is utilized to excise a donor ellipse from the posterior scalp. This technique maximizes the amount of hair harvested while minimizing scarring. The elliptical excision can be performed using a single-blade or a double-blade knife with spacers in between (Fig. 3.3). It can also be performed utilizing the donor dissection technique, a process by which excellent hemostasis is maintained so hair follicles are directly visualized during the harvesting process, which minimizes the transection rate. A series of 50 hair transplant patients where the donor dissection technique was utilized resulted in a 1.9% transection rate during the harvesting process.[8] We utilize skin hooks on both sides of the ellipse for optimal visibility (Fig. 3.4A). The incision should be below the follicle bulbs into the subcutaneous tissue to minimize transection of hair follicles. The ellipse is removed just below the bulbs with scissors or a scalpel (Fig. 3.4B).[3]

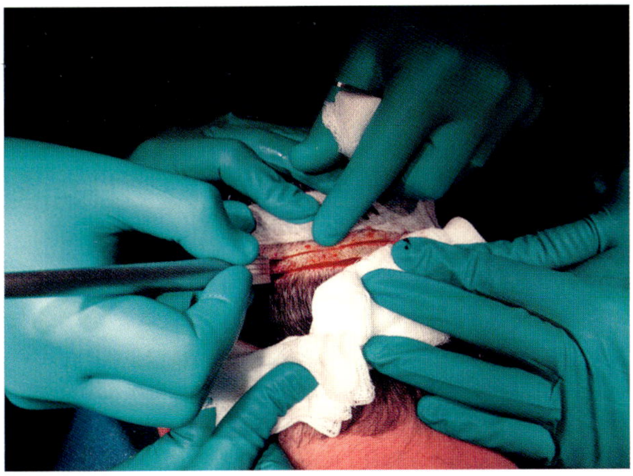

Fig. 3.3: Elliptical donor strip harvesting with a double-blade knife with spacer.

In general, donor strips should not be >1 cm wide, as strips >1 cm in width have a greater risk of poor healing, hypertrophic scars, and widened scars. The length of the donor ellipse depends on the number of grafts needed for the surgery. In general, the average patient has 65–85 follicular groupings per square centimeter and the length of the elliptical excision can be calculated based on the average density of the donor area and number of hairs needed for the surgery.[4,9] *See* Table 3.1 for a guide to predict donor strip size based on the available donor density.[3]

Once the strip is harvested, the donor region must be repaired with staples or sutures (Fig. 3.5). A two-layered closure is typically not needed, but may be used when the site is under tension. Some transplant surgeons use a closure technique known as "trichophytic closure", where a narrow rim of epidermis on the inferior border of the ellipse is removed so the underlying hairs grow directly into and better conceal the scar. This may improve the appearance of the scar but may also result in slightly higher rates of cyst or ingrown hair formation.[3] Once the suturing or stapling is complete, a temporary dressing of Aquaphor, a nonstick dressing such as Tefla, and an elastic bandage is used to create a pressure dressing (Figs. 3.6A and B). A winter beanie or a summer scarf is then placed, and stays on the patient's head until the next day.

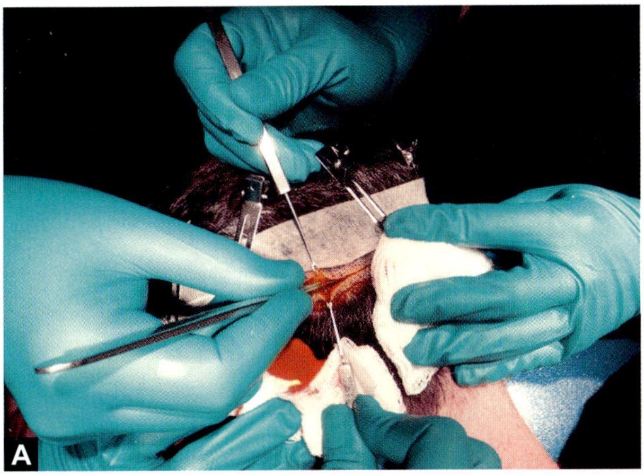

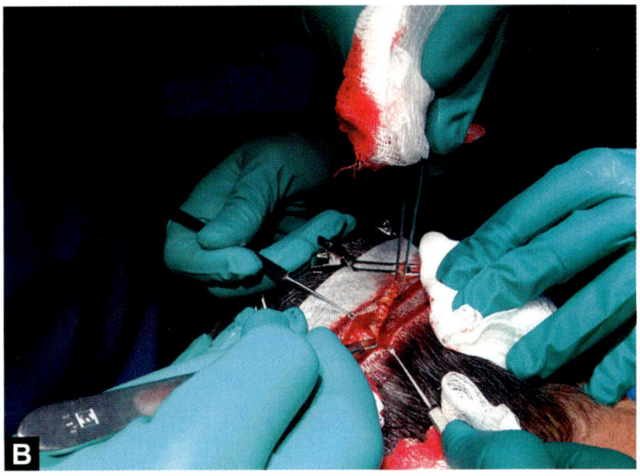

Figs. 3.4A and B: (A) Skin hooks to maximize visibility. (B) Removing ellipse just below bulbs to minimize transection.

Key points to emphasize to the patient include: that after elliptical donor harvesting, there is no change in the perceived density of hair in the donor region, a permanent linear scar will be visible in the posterior scalp if the hair is shaved or closely cut (Fig. 3.7), there is a limited amount of donor hair, and that transplanted hair from the donor area will grow for as long as it is generically programmed to grow once transplanted (for most patients this is lifelong).[3]

Table 3.1: Predicting donor strip size based on donor density.

Donor density (follicular units per cm²)	*Strip size required to harvest 1,000 follicular units*
Above average > 85	12 × 0.8 cm
Average 65–85	15 × 0.8 cm
Below average < 50	22 × 0.8 cm

Source: Adapted from Avram M, Rogers N. Contemporary hair transplantation. Dermatol Surg. 2009;35(11):1705-19.

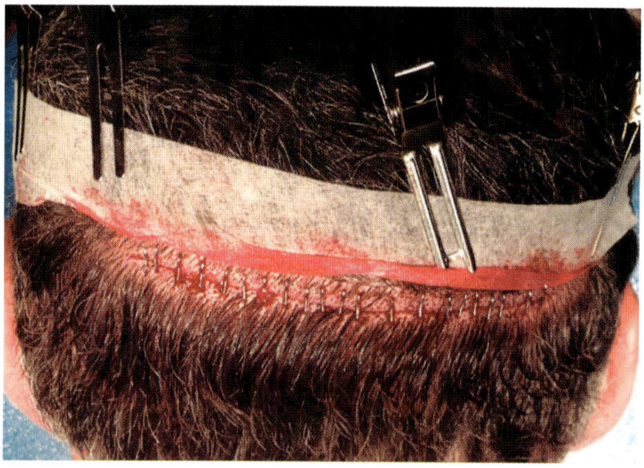

Fig. 3.5: Donor region repaired with staples.

Due to stretching of the scalp, it is thought that at least two to three elliptical separate excisions of 1 cm in width can be taken from the posterior scalp without difficulty with closure. In general, the maximum width of elliptical donor harvesting is determined by the amount of scalp laxity present in a patient. Depending on donor laxity, a safe strip width is generally 10–25 mm.[10] There are many ways to predict donor site laxity. One method is to squeeze the scalp between your fingers. This is a subjective test and relies on experience, but for an experienced surgeon, it is often quite reliable.[10] In general, lateral donor areas have less laxity, afford less camouflage, and yield few grafts.

There is also formula developed by Mayer and Pauls that can be used to determine scalp elasticity. With this method, a 50 mm line is marked on the occipital donor area, and the borders are squeezed together along the horizontal axis. The formula is:

Scalp elasticity = $(50\ \text{mm} - x)\ (100\%)/50\ \text{mm}$, where x is the length of the compressed skin segment in millimeter.

Mayer and Pauls[11] used this formula to determine scalp elasticity in 400 patients. They found the range of scalp elasticity in these patients was between 10% and 45%, with an average of 24%. They concluded that a 10% elasticity represented a tight scalp and a 45% elasticity represented a very elastic scalp. They suggested that scalps with low elasticity (10% elasticity) may yield a 5 mm strip, a scalp with average elasticity (24%) may yield a 12 mm strip, and a very loose scalp (45% elasticity) may yield a 22.5 mm strip.[10,11]

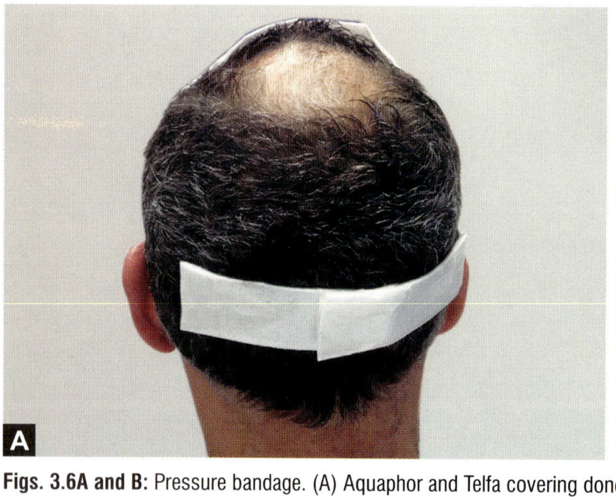

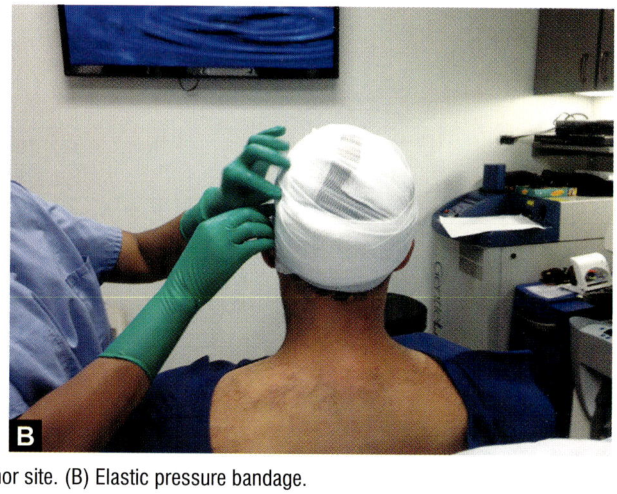

Figs. 3.6A and B: Pressure bandage. (A) Aquaphor and Telfa covering donor site. (B) Elastic pressure bandage.

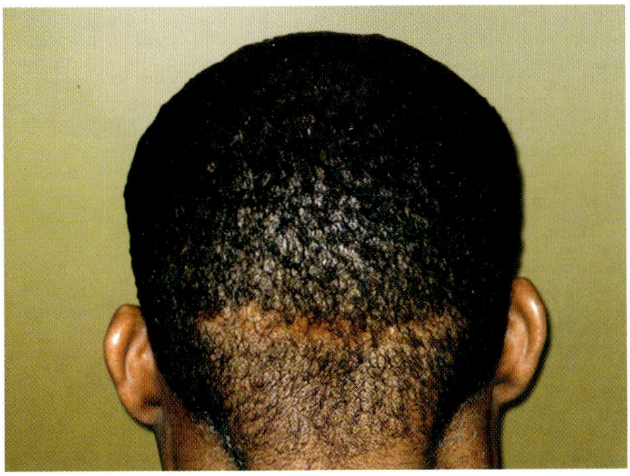

Fig. 3.7: Linear scar after elliptical donor harvesting.

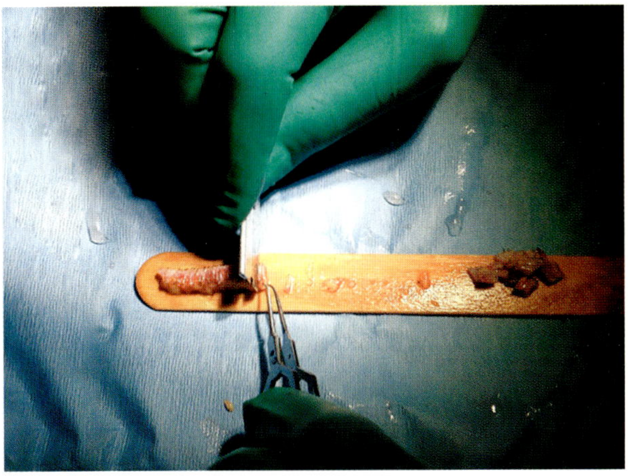

Fig. 3.8: Slivering of the strip.

Some hair transplant surgeons also feel that preoperative scalp massage can be used to increase scalp laxity. The results vary, but patients can be instructed to massage the scalp in a vertical fashion for 3–5 minutes multiple time during the day for 2–4 weeks prior to the procedure.[10]

PROCESSING OF THE ELLIPSE INTO FOLLICULAR UNITS

After the donor strip is removed, it takes about 45–60 minutes for three to four experienced assistants to process the strip into 1,000–1,5000 follicular units.[4] First, the strip is divided into slivers, much like slicing a loaf of bread (Fig. 3.8). Then, each sliver is divided into individual follicular units of one to four hair grafts, depending on their natural groupings in the scalp (Fig. 3.9). Microscopes are often used for increased precision. The technique of donor dissection with direct visualization of hair follicles is also often used to decrease transection rates during the graft cutting process. A paper by Pathomvanich reports the transection rate during graft cutting was reduced to 1.2% using the donor dissection technique.[8]

FOLLICULAR UNIT EXTRACTION

The concept of FUE was introduced in the early 21st century and has been refined over the past decade. There are many devices designed for FUE. They range from manual to powered, sharp and dull devices. We will briefly review some of the more common devices used for FUE in the following section.

The main advantage of over traditional elliptical excision is the absence of a linear scar. Follicular unit

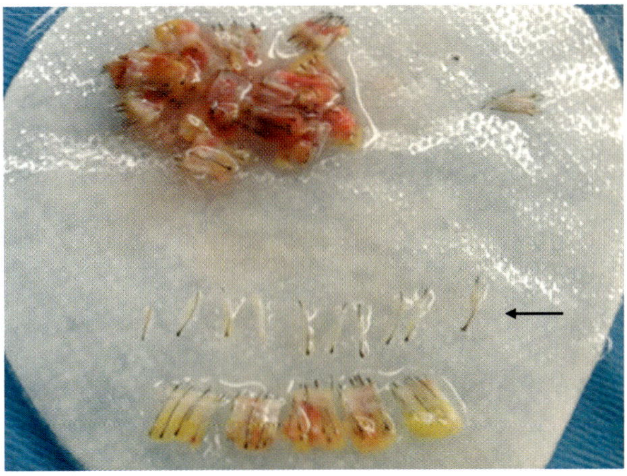

Fig. 3.9: Follicular units obtained via elliptical donor harvesting (arrow). Above and below, the slivers are pictured.

extraction is also less invasive than traditional donor strip excision, and has less downtime involved in the recovery process. If the donor area is overharvested by FUE, however, it is possible that the donor site can have a moth-eaten or pseudosyphilitic appearance. *See* Table 3.2 for a comparison of standard ellipse versus FUE donor harvesting.[3,12]

MANUAL FUE

Rassman et al. described a technique of manual FUE known as the Fox Procedure, utilizing a 1 mm punch biopsy placed directly over an individual follicular unit, following the angle of emerging hairs, until the punch is passed partially through the dermis. Once the initial advancement is made, the bulk of the follicle is pulled with forceps, extracting the follicular unit from the scalp. They also describe the Fox Test, which can be used to determine which patients are good

Table 3.2: A comparison of standard ellipse to FUE harvesting.

	Standard ellipse	*Follicular unit extraction*
Scarring	Linear scar	No linear scar
Time to harvest grafts	10–20 minutes for 300–2,000	Manual FUE 1 hour: 100–200 grafts (operator dependent) Powered FUE: Operator and device dependent ARTAS robotic FUE 45–60 minutes: 300–600 grafts 60–120 minutes: 600–1,200 grafts
Healing time	7–10 days	3–5 days
Cost	Minimal	Manual FUE: Minimal Powered FUE: Device dependent ARTAS robotic FUE: Significant to purchase machine and per surgery fee
Transection rate	Low with experienced team Widely variable with inexperienced team	Manual FUE: Operator dependent Powered FUE: Operator dependent ARTAS robotic FUE: Low to low-moderate
Physician skill	Standard skin excision techniques	Manual and powered FUE: Technically demanding, operator dependent ARTAS robotic FUE: Knowledge of software program and robot
Technician skill	Skilled technician mandatory to create follicular units with low transection	Skilled technician needed to remove grafts from scalp and assess quality under magnification before placing in recipient site
Reliability	Technician + physician dependent	Manual FUE: Technician + physician dependent Powered and ARTAS robotic FUE: Technician + physician + robot dependent
Area of donor site shaved	1.5 cm × 8–10 cm	4–8 cm × 10–20 cm

(FUE: Follicular unit extraction).
Source: Adapted from Avram MR, Watkins SA. Robotic follicular unit extraction in hair transplantation. Dermatol Surg. 2014;4(12):1319-27.

candidates for the procedure. In the Fox Test, at least five follicular units are extracted from the back of the scalp using the FOX Procedure. The extracted grafts are examined under a microscope for their integrity and/or sent for histologic examination. Then a score of 1–5 is given to the patient that predicts whether or not the patient is a good candidate for manual FUE. A score of 1 was assigned if all the follicular units extracted were intact, a score of 2 was assigned to those patients who had all grafts with most of the anatomy intact, but a loss of fat around the lower part of the follicle or some degree of amputation in <20% of the follicular units, and a score of 4 was given when most of the surrounding fat was avulsed with a significant number of follicles amputated, a score of 5 reflected significant damage in all of the grafts. Patients who scored a 1 or 2 in the Fox Test were considered good candidates for the procedure, class 3 were neutral, and class 4 or 5 were not considered candidates for the Fox Procedure.[13] Figure 3.10 shows an example of a manual and a motorized FUE device.

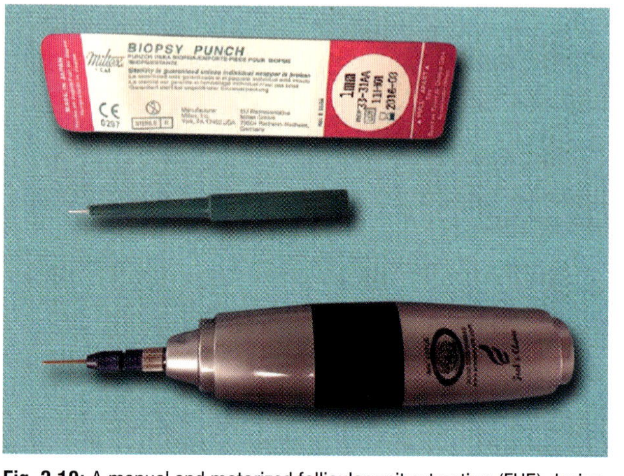

Fig. 3.10: A manual and motorized follicular unit extraction (FUE) device. Motorized FUE device pictured at bottom.

Powered Manual FUE Devices

There are several motorized FUE devices on the market. We will discuss two of the most well-known devices below, the SAFE system and the Neograft.

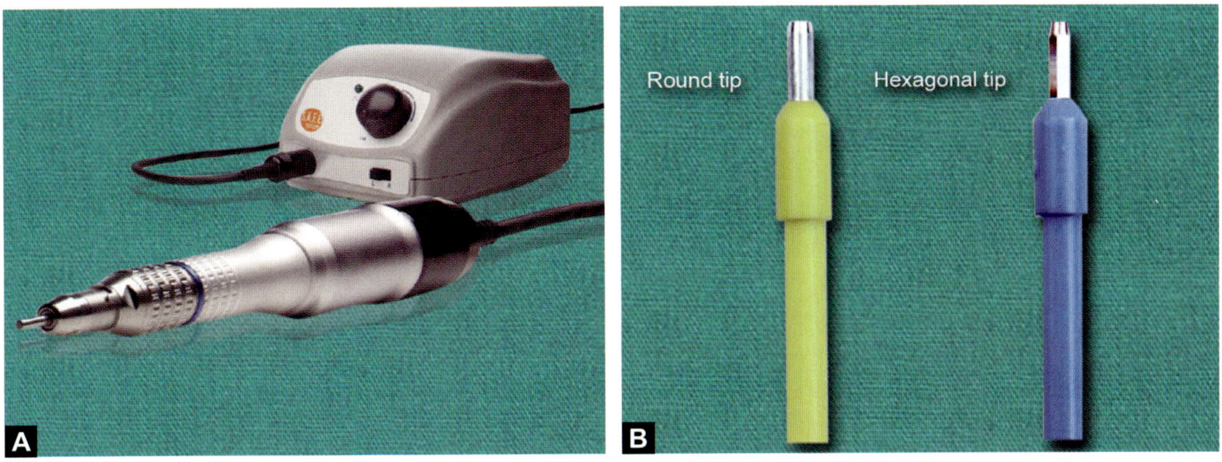

Figs. 3.11A and B: (A) The SAFE system. Image courtesy of Dr. James Harris. www.hsccolorado.com. (B) Standard Round and Hexagonal tips used with the SAFE system.

SAFE System

The surgically advanced follicular extraction (SAFE) system (Fig. 3.11A) is a powered FUE device invented by James Harris. It is a motorized device that uses either cylindrical ("round") or hexagonal ("Hex") blunt tip punches for graft dissection (Fig. 3.11B). The punches come in .8, .9, 1.0, and 1.2 mm sizes. The principle advantage of the blunt punch dissection technique is the ability to dissect to the depth of 4mm with minimal transection of follicles. The average depth of dissection for sharp punch systems is 2–2.5 mm. Harris reports that a deeper depth of dissection means less force is required to remove the graft from the skin, and therefore less trauma to the grafts. The latest innovation, the hexagonal tip, induces a small amount of vibration which helps separate the surrounding tissue from follicular units further, leading to even lower transection rates. The isolated follicular units are then removed with forceps and evaluated for integrity prior to transplantation.

James Harris reports the SAFE system has expanded patient candidacy to include blacks and some of the patients who are classified as not eligible for FUE by the Fox Test proposed by Rassman and colleagues.[13,14] Based on a series of 59 patients from whom 6,947 grafts were harvested, Harris reports an average of 6.14% transection rate (range 1.7–15%) with the SAFE system. The only adverse reactions reported were two buried grafts resulting in inflammatory subcutaneous cysts requiring excision. He concludes that the SAFE system provides methodology and instrumentation that can enhance FUE techniques and expand patient candidacy.[14] Like manual FUE, however, this method of FUE is user dependent as it requires technical skill to perform with speed and accuracy.

Neograft

The Neograft machine is a powered, handheld surgical device that utilizes a sharp punch biopsy to extract individual follicular units from the donor area. It is operator dependent, as an operator guides and selects which hair follicles are to be harvested. It then uses a controlled pneumatic pressure system to remove the graft from the donor area and stores grafts in a saline filled canister until the grafts are ready for implantation in the recipient site. Compared with the ARTAS robotic system, the Neograft relies on operator skill and experience to determine which grafts and at which angle grafts should be harvested, while the ARTAS robotic system relies on computerized digital imaging to concisely harvest grafts.[15,16]

● ROBOTIC SYSTEM

ARTAS Robotic System

The ARTAS robotic system (Restoration Robotics, Inc, San Jose, CA) is the only truly robotic system for FUE on the market to date (Fig. 3.12). It was Food and Drug Administration approved for hair transplantation in 2011. A 1 mm punch is attached to the robotic arm consisting of a "needle-within-needle," where the sharp inner punch is surrounded by a blunt outer punch. The sharp inner punch creates a shallow 1 mm incision and the blunt outer punch spinning at 400–800 rpm subsequently dissects deeper and

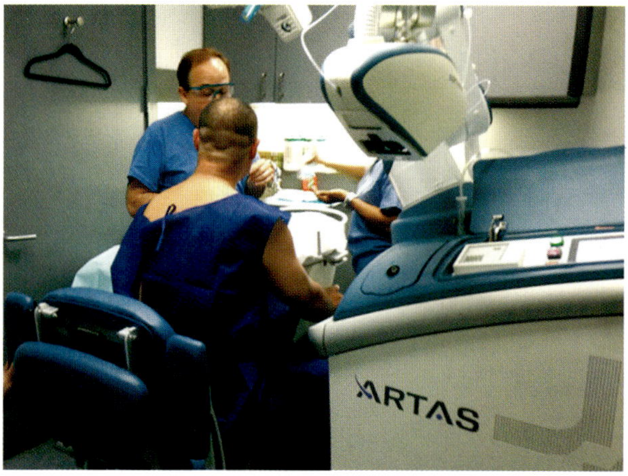

Fig. 3.12: ARTAS robotic system.

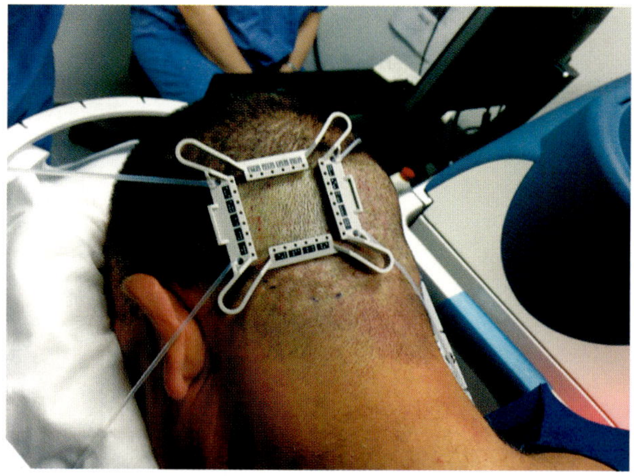

Fig. 3.13: Grid for harvesting with ARTAS device.

separates the follicular unit from the surrounding tissue. A suction system then elevates the follicular unit from surrounding skin, making it easier to manually extract the graft. A combination of stereoscopic cameras managed by image processing software allows the sharp and blunt punches to identify the precise angle and direction of hair growth. This continuous imaging feedback allows the robot to accurately harvest each follicular grouping. The sensors work by detecting the pigment in hair follicles, so if a patient has white or blonde hair, the donor hair must be dyed brown or black prior to harvesting. This is typically done with a temporary hair dye immediately prior to the procedure. Hairs must also be trimmed to 1–2 mm in length for the digital imaging system to function properly, and a plastic grid with fiducials (appear like dominos) to calibrate the system must be placed and moved on the scalp to facilitate donor harvesting (Fig. 3.13). Due to the high level of automation, the robot can remove 400–600 grafts per hour. There is a minimum distance of 1.6 mm between extracted follicular groupings to minimize the risk of overharvesting the donor area. Once the follicular units are harvested, they are inspected by experienced technicians who trim excess tissue off the grafts prior to implantation of the hairs in the recipient site.[17] Figure 3.14 for an example of typical grafts harvested by the ARTS robotic device.

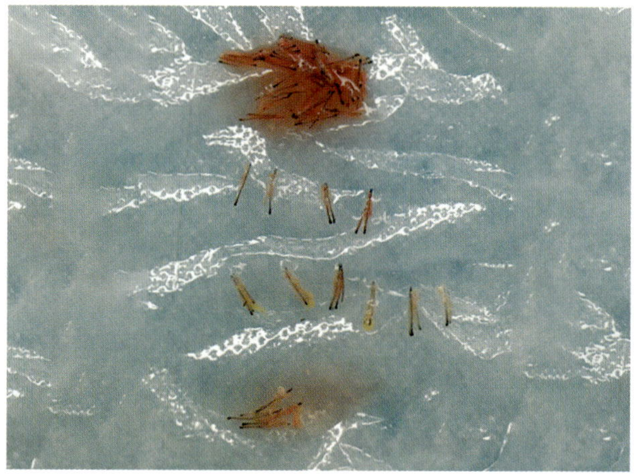

Fig. 3.14: Typical follicular unit extraction grafts harvested with ARTAS device.

WOUND CARE AFTER DONOR HARVESTING

After the hair transplant procedure is complete whether donor harvesting is done via an FUE or elliptical excision, a pressure bandage is placed on the scalp as described above. We recommend the patient keep the pressure bandage in place until the day after the procedure. Beginning postoperative day 1, we recommend the patient wash the donor site with soap and water and apply Aquaphor ointment twice daily for the next 7 days. Wound care is the same for both FUE and elliptical donor harvesting. Typically, the FUE donor sites heal within 3–5 days and patients can resume their regular activities. With elliptical donor harvesting, however, we remove the sutures at day 7 and ask patients to avoid heavy exercise at least until the sutures are removed.

If the patient is diabetic and at an increased risk of infection, we typically prescribe Bactroban (mupirocin) ointment to be applied twice daily to the donor site instead of the usual Aquaphor. Oral antibiotics are not routinely given.

REFERENCES

1. Orentreich N. Autografts in alopecias and other selected dermatological conditions. Ann NY Acad Sci. 1959;83:463-79.
2. Park JH, Na YC, Moh JS, et al. Predicting the permanent safe donor area for hair transplantation in Koreans with male pattern baldness according to the position of the parietal whorl. Arch Plast Surg. 2014;41(3):277-84.
3. Avram M, Rogers N. Contemporary hair transplantation. Dermatol Surg. 2009;35(11):1705-19.
4. Avram MR. Hair transplantation: new concepts in 2005. J Cosmet Laser Ther. 2005;7(2):77-80.
5. Bisaccia E, Scarborough D. Hair transplant by incisional strip harvesting. J Dermatol Surg Oncol. 1994; 20(7):443-8.
6. Knudsen RG. The donor area. Facial Plast Surg Clin North Am. 2004;12(2):233-40.
7. Rassman WR, Carson S. Micrografting in extensive quantities. The ideal hair restoration procedure. Dermatol Surg. 1995;21(4):306-11.
8. Pathomvanich D. Donor harvesting: a new approach to minimize transection of hair follicles. Dermatol Surg. 2000;26(4):345-8.
9. Jimenez F, Ruifernandez JM. Distribution of human hair in follicular units. A mathematical model for estimating the donor size in follicular unit transplantation. Dermatol Surg. 1999;25(4):294-8.
10. Buchwach KA. Graft harvesting and management of the donor site. Facial Plast Surg Clin North Am. 2013;21(3):363-74.
11. Mayer M, Pauls T. Scalp elasticity scale. Hair Transplant Forum Intl. 2005;15:122-23.
12. Avram MR, Watkins SA. Robotic follicular unit extraction in hair transplantation. Dermatol Surg. 2014;40(12):1319-27.
13. Rassman WR, Bernstein RM, McClellan R, et al. Follicular unit extraction: minimally invasive surgery for hair transplantation. Dermatol Surg. 2002;28(8): 720-28.
14. Harris JA. New methodology and instrumentation for follicular unit extraction: lower follicle transection rates and expanded patient candidacy. Dermatol Surg. 2006;32(1):56-61; discussion 61-2.
15. Available from www.neograft.com.
16. Available from www.restorationrobotics.com.
17. Rose PT, Nusbaum B. Robotic hair restoration. Dermatol Clin. 2014;32(1):97-107.

CHAPTER

4

Hairline Design/Holding Solutions/Graft Creation

Francisco Jimenez-Acosta

HAIRLINE DESIGN

The single and most important aspect to achieve a natural appearance to the hair transplant is the creation of the anterior hairline design. This is accomplished through the appropriate location of a few landmarks that help to design the hairline as well as the use of a large number of small grafts [one and two hair follicular units (FUs)].

The equipment needed for hairline design is simply a marking pen, a ruler, alcohol swabs (to remove markings), and a handheld mirror. I recommend the use of a ruler specifically made for hairline design known as an Assist to Hairline Design (Cole Instruments, Alpharetta, GA), because it has several vertical scales and horizontal and vertical reference lines that allow the surgeon to take hairline measurements at different levels of the forehead to ensure the symmetry of the hairline[1] (Figs. 4.1A and B). More sophisticated devices to assist in the hairline such as the Pathomvanich laser device can also be used for this purpose.[2]

Landmarks for Creating a Natural Frontal Hairline

The first thing to do is to draw the landmarks that establish the height and shape of the frontal hairline. These landmarks are only guidelines to determine the hairline placement and have to be individualized depending on the size and shape of the head and the degree of alopecia.

- *Midfrontal point (MFP)*: The first landmark that needs to be drawn is the MFP, which is the most anterior point of the frontal hairline (Fig. 4.2). In

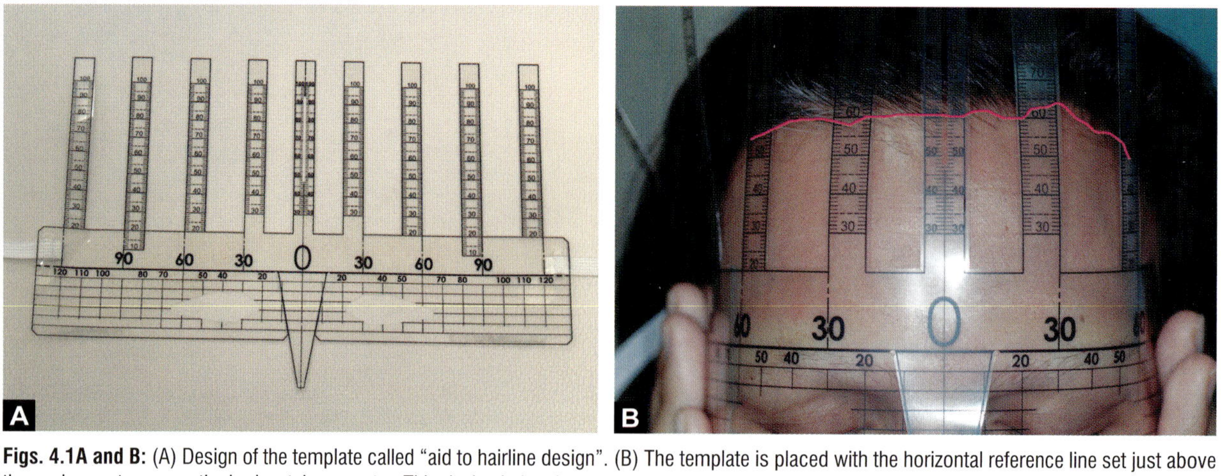

Figs. 4.1A and B: (A) Design of the template called "aid to hairline design". (B) The template is placed with the horizontal reference line set just above the eyebrows to ensure the horizontal symmetry. This device helps the surgeon to measure the height of the hairline and its symmetry.

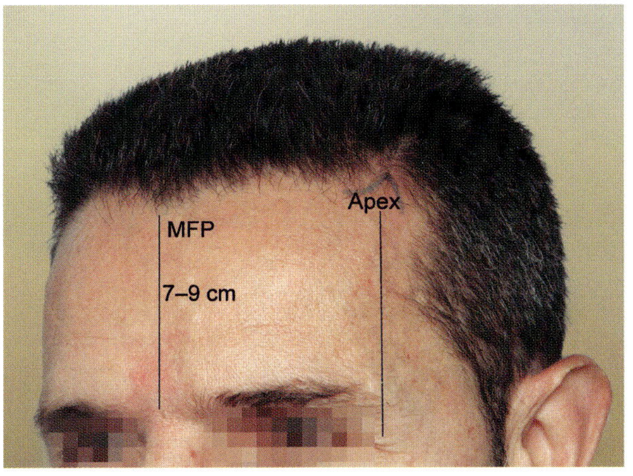

Fig. 4.2: The midfrontal point (MFP) is the anterior-most point of the frontal hairline, and in most male patients, the MFP is located between 7 and 9 cm above the glabella. The apex is where the frontal hairline meets the temporal hair.

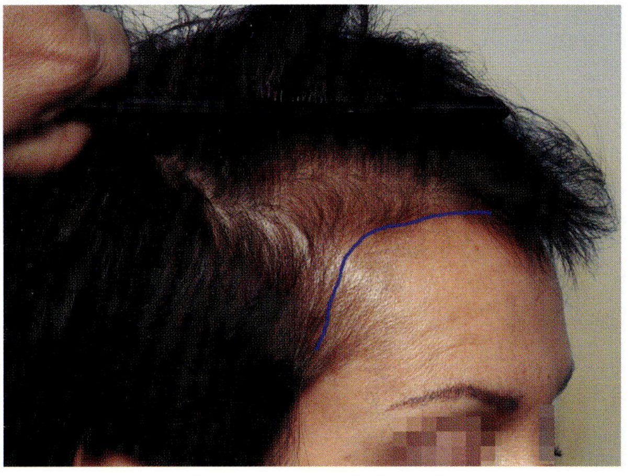

Fig. 4.3: In females, the hairline can be designed following a rounded shape with no temporal recessions.

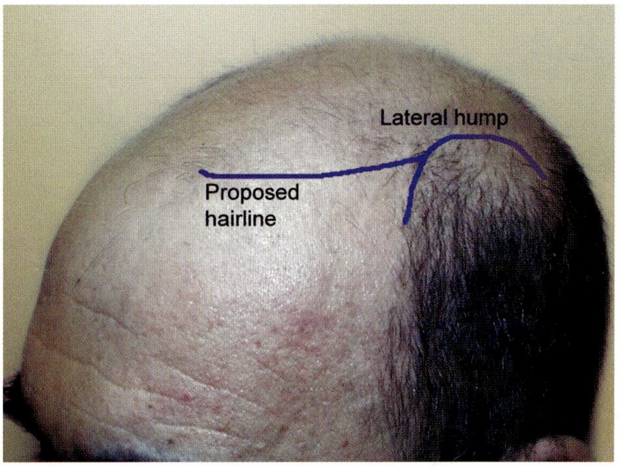

Fig. 4.4: Lifting the temporoparietal fringe with the use of "lateral humps" helps to design the frontal hairline in its proper position.

most male patients, the MFP is located between 7 and 9 cm above the glabella. In extreme balding, it is preferable to make the MFP a little higher, at about 10–12 cm from the glabella in order to conserve donor hair. In females, the MFP is lower than in males, normally at 6–7 cm.[3]

- *Frontotemporal point (FTP; the apex)*: This should be the next point to be drawn. This point is located where a vertical line upward from the lateral canthus of the eye meets any remaining temporal hair (Fig. 4.2). A gently curving hairline should be drawn joining the MFP with the two FTPs. In males, it is important to always maintain a significant frontotemporal recession. As a general rule, the apex must never be lower than the MFP, as this creates a feminized hairline. The problem in advanced balding is that the parietal border might be so low that it does not allow creation of an aesthetic FTP. In this circumstance, we first have to raise the parietal border by creating so-called lateral humps, which enable proper design of an FTP. In females, the hairline requires a design that includes a more rounded temporal infill and a lower hairline than that created for males (Fig. 4.3).
- *Lateral (parietal) humps:* The lateral hump is the superior extension of the inferiorly directed hair of the temporoparietal fringe (Fig. 4.4). This landmark is important because it represents the lateral extent of the anterior hairline (AHL).[4]
- *Transition zone:* The hairlines should be designed with a 5–10 mm wide transition zone that merges the bald forehead to a zone of increasing gradient of density. This transition zone is where most single hair grafts are placed (Fig. 4.5). The transition zone should be created with irregularities to mimic a natural hairline.
- *Irregularities of the hairline:* As an absolute rule, hairlines should never be flat, but broken up with irregularities. They are normally created using triangular clusters of hairs and gaps. These triangles are of varying depth and width (Fig. 4.6). The more irregularities we create in the hairline, the more natural it appears (Figs. 4.7A and B).

Landmarks for Creating the Temporal Triangles

Restoration of the temporal triangle is performed according to the personal preferences of patient and surgeon. The temple is difficult to recreate and there is no need to do it unless the patient asks for

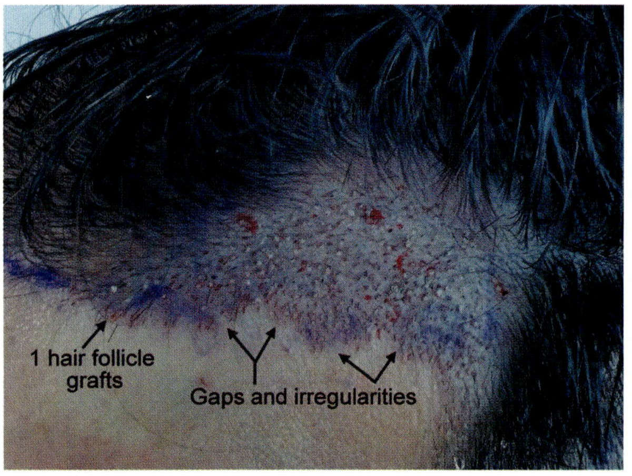

Fig. 4.5: Transition zone. The first 5 mm of the anterior hairline consists of one hair follicular unit grafts. Note the irregularities and gaps created in the hairline (arrows).

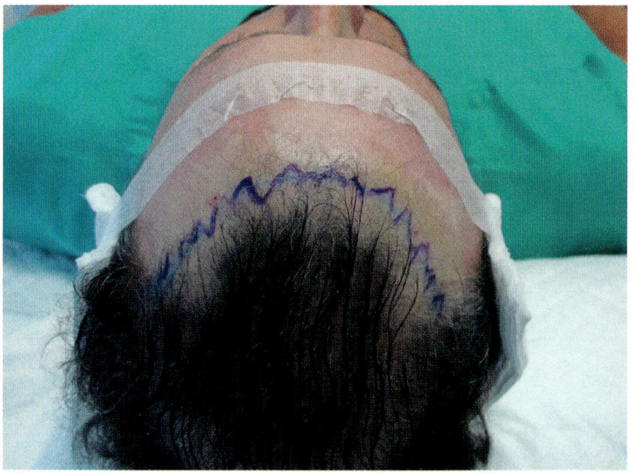

Fig. 4.6: The anterior hairline should not be flat. Always make it irregular but symmetrical.

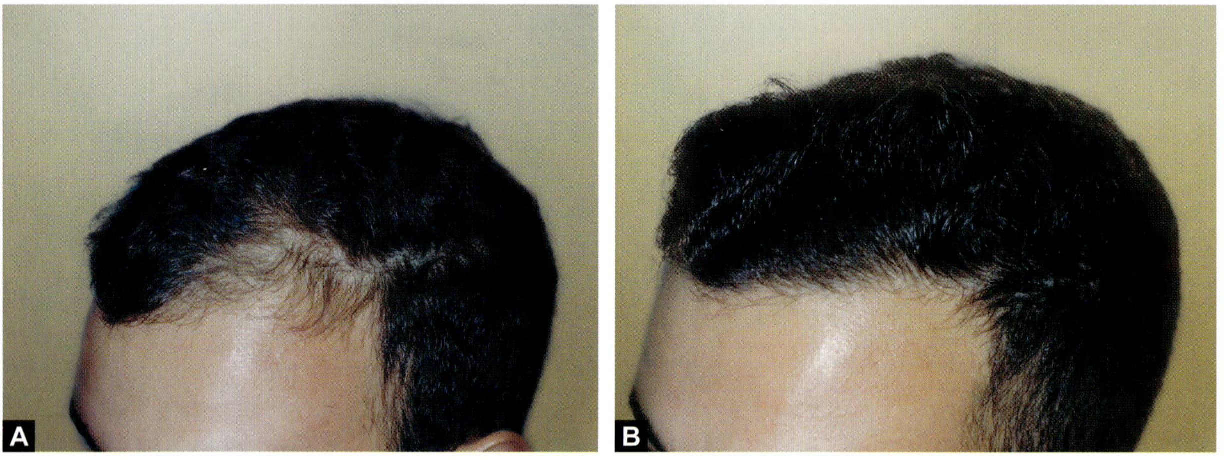

Figs. 4.7A and B: Patient Norwood type 2 before and after hair transplantation. This case shows that the transplanted hairline should look completely natural if two basic principles are followed: Only use single hair grafts in the anterior-most hairline and create irregularities.

it and is conscious about its loss. The first landmark that should be located and drawn is the temporal point (TP) (Fig. 4.8). Many times, the identification of existing residual terminal or vellus hairs is sufficient to correctly locate the TPs. However, if the TPs are entirely absent, they are best located by the drawing of two lines[5]:

1. One line goes approximately from the "crus of helix" of the ear lobe to the MFP.
2. The second line goes from the tip of the nose through the pupil of the eye and intersects the first line.

We have to make sure that when placing the hairs in the temporal triangle, the hair exits at an acute angle in a posterior direction. The safest thing is to follow the direction of the existing hair. Grading of the single hairs to place the finest hairs at the anterior border will allow the most natural result. Two hair grafts can be placed more posteriorly in the temple.

The Parietal-Vertex Posterior Transition Zone

This zone indicates the posterior border of the parietal scalp, where the vertex starts. In this zone, the shape of the scalp changes from the horizontal plane of the parietal scalp to the more vertical plane of the vertex and occipital scalp. In many severe balding patients, the goal is to first complete the placement of grafts in the frontal and parietal scalp ending in this transition zone. This zone is called "transition zone" because the grafts should not create a posterior wall, but as mentioned before in the transition frontal zone, the grafts should be placed creating an irregular line with

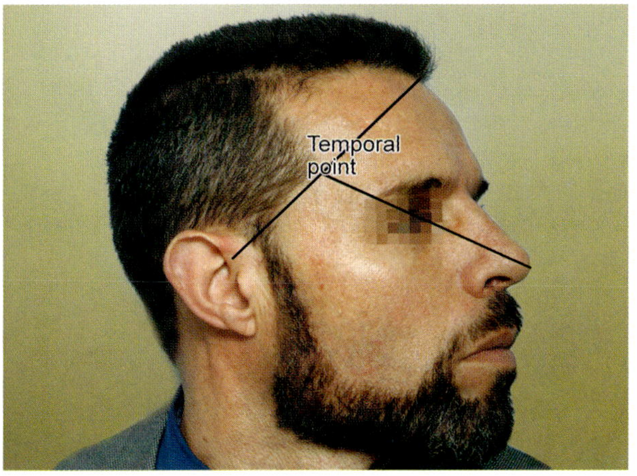

Fig. 4.8: Location of the temporal point. This point can be found by the intersection of two lines: a line from the "crus of helix" of the ear to the mid-frontal point and a line from the tip of the nose through the pupil of the eye.

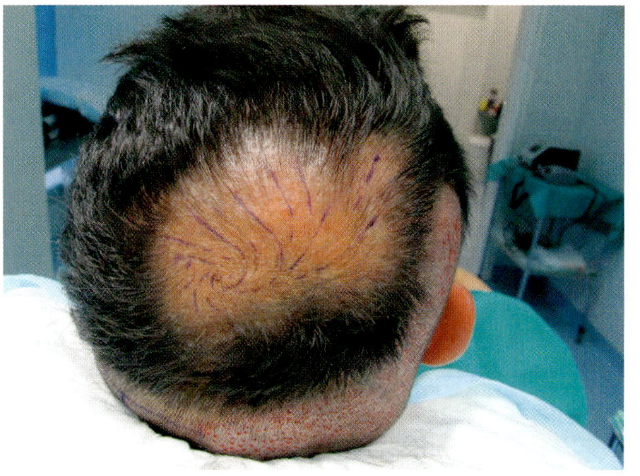

Fig. 4.9: In hair restoration of the vertex region, it is important to follow the direction of the fine existing hairs and recreate the original swirl pattern.

a transition of density and placing also numerous single hairs in the most posterior part of this transition zone. This will help to recreate the naturalness of this zone.

The Vertex

The key to recreating the vertex is to identify and follow the direction of the hair swirls. The vertex may have one or two swirls, on the right or left side. The existing miniaturized hairs are very helpful for identifying the swirl and lines should be drawn following the changes in the direction of the hair (Fig. 4.9).

The vertex usually needs more hair than one would expect. So, the vertex should be filled when the transplant on the frontal and parietal scalp has been completed and if the patient still has enough donor hair remaining.

Key Points to Follow in Creating the Hairline

1. The hairline should be placed in a conservative location so that it will look natural as the patient ages and continues to lose hair.
2. Measure the hairline with the ruler as much as possible, but then take a step back and make sure it looks correct.
3. In males, never draw the MFP <7 cm from the glabella.
4. Never chase the receding temporoparietal fringe with the hairline; instead, build up the "parietal humps".
5. Remember you can always lower the hairline in a subsequent session, but hairlines cannot be raised.
6. In males, try to maintain a significant frontotemporal recession.
7. You can never create too many microirregularities in the frontal hairline.
8. The direction and acute angle of the hair are an important consideration in restoring the temporal triangles.

HOLDING SOLUTIONS

Any topic related to maneuvers that can enhance hair graft survival is of considerable interest for hair transplant surgeons. For this reason, holding solutions are currently a hot topic in hair transplant meetings.

During the course of a hair transplantation procedure, the cells and/or tissues experience multiple forms of stresses related to the procedure from before extraction of the donor area, through the dissection and past the point of reimplantation. Once the donor strip is removed [or once the FU is removed in the case of follicular unit extraction (FUE)], the cells within the tissue are immediately cut off from their supply of oxygen, glucose, and other necessary nutrients. During this ischemic phase, the donor hair is maintained in petri dishes filled with a solution (holding solution) to keep the grafts hydrated. In the strip harvesting technique, these hair grafts may be kept in the holding solution an average of 3–6 hours (depending on the speed of the cutting process and the length of the session). In the FUE technique, the grafts are also kept in holding solutions until implantation, but the length of time may vary because the hair surgeon might decide to start implantation after, e.g. 500 extractions and then continue with the extractions or to begin after all the FUs have been extracted. In any case, the time that the hair graft is left out of the body in the holding solution until it is implanted is a critical factor for hair growth survival. In a classical research study, Limmer[6] showed that survival of grafts stored in chilled saline decreases with the length of time between removal from the donor site and implantation in the recipient sites. Limmer showed that the survival rate is high if the FUs are transplanted in <6 hours (95% at 2 hours and 86% at 6 hours between harvest and transplantation), but that it fell significantly after that timeframe.

The most common holding solutions used among hair transplant surgeons are normal saline and Ringer's lactate because they are intravenous solutions that are cheap and easily available and because their successful use has been observed over a period of decades.[7] However, it is worth considering how saline lacks many of the key elements of an ideal holding solution: (1) correct osmolarity, (2) correct pH and buffering capability, (3) antioxidants, and (4) nutrients. For this reason, other holding solutions that include additives that work as energy sources and antioxidants could in theory be more beneficial. These include culture media-based solutions like Williams E, multiple electrolyte solutions like Plasma-Lyte A, or intracellular-type solutions like Hypothermosol. Unfortunately, the lack of evidence-based studies means no conclusion can be made as to the best holding solution for hair transplantation. Platelet-rich plasma (PRP) containing numerous growth factors such as platelet-derived growth factor or vascular endothelial growth factor has been reported to improved survival of hair grafts when added to the holding solution.[8] However, to date, the use of PRP in hair restoration surgery is still controversial and no standard protocols have as yet been established.

Temperature is thought to be a factor that may influence graft survival. At low temperatures, the oxygen and energy demand of the grafts falls as metabolic activity is reduced. However, a cold temperature can also injure the grafts by perturbations in osmoregulation and intracellular acidosis. In this situation, an intracellular-like solution, as opposed to an isotonic/extracellular-like solution such as culture media or saline, would be more suitable to balance the altered cellular ion concentrations that result from hypothermic temperatures.[9] The current perception is that if the grafts are to be kept out of the body for < 6 hours, they can be left at room temperature with no difference in the survival rate than at chilling storage (1–4°C). For long sessions lasting over 12 hours or on those rare occasions when the surgeon needs to store the grafts overnight in a standard refrigerator, an intracellular-like solution such as Hypothermol-FRS has been shown to be an ideal environment for the grafts.[10]

Adenosine triphosphate *(ATP)*: When a hair follicle is transplanted, the grafts can take from 3 to 5 days to be reconnected to their own blood supply. During this time the follicle graft is ischemic, resulting in decreased production of the cell's refined fuel ATP. Adenosine triphosphate driven cell membrane pumps maintain the osmolarity balance of the cell. The addition to the holding solution of a recently commercialized liposomal ATP solution has been proposed in order to counterbalance the ischemic environment that the grafts endure after removal from the donor scalp. Liposomal ATP has the capacity to efficiently deliver ATP into the cells by fusing the lipid membrane of the liposomes with the cells' own lipid membranes. Protocols for use of liposomal ATP are based on personal experience, and further studies are needed to evaluate its real impact on graft survival. When using ATP as an additive for the holding solutions, 1–10 cc of the concentrated ATP can be added to 100 cc of holding solution. When used as a postoperative solution, the current recommendation is to add 10 cc of concentrated ATP to 90 cc of saline in a spray bottle and have the patients spray the solution in the recipient area every 2 hours for the first 48 hours and then every 4 hours thereafter for a further 2–3 days.[10]

GRAFT CREATION

Strip Harvesting with Microscopic Dissection of the Grafts

Once the donor tissue has been harvested, the donor strip is immediately immersed in the holding solution and given to the technician to cut into slivers.

Instruments Used for Graft Creation

Graft preparation is performed immediately using stereomicroscopes and microsurgical instrumentation. Stereomicroscopes are the gold standard for FU graft preparation (Fig. 4.10). They offer the proper magnification and have an excellent light source. There are several brands that are popular for hair

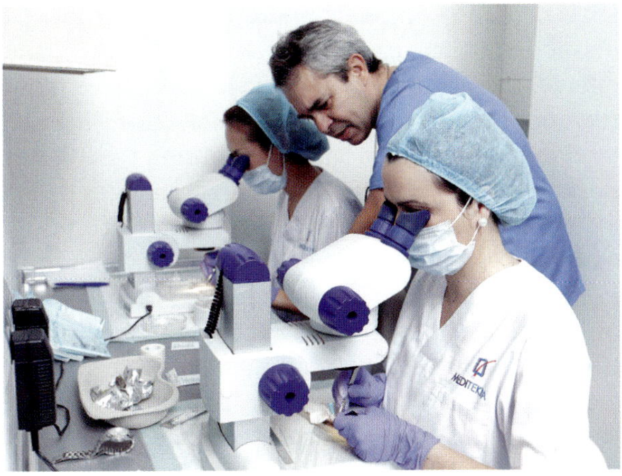

Fig. 4.10: Technicians using Zeiss stereomicroscopes for microscopic dissection of the follicular units. The surgeon supervises the process.

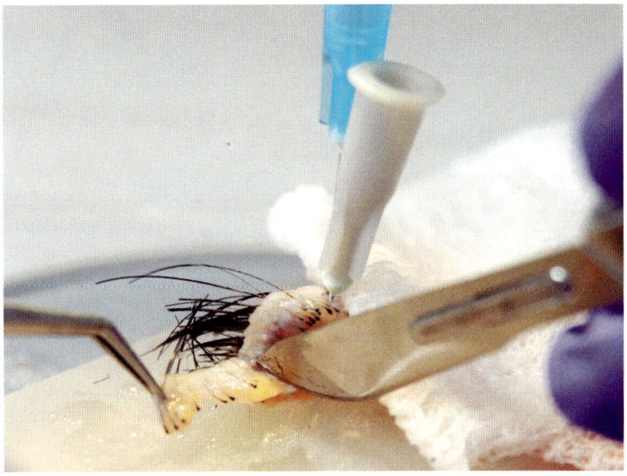

Fig. 4.11: Slivers are created from the donor strip using #10 blades. Ideally, the sliver should be thin (one follicular unit thin) to facilitate the dissection of the follicular unit grafts.

transplantation including Zeiss, Mantis, Meiji, Nikon, and Motic. Most assistant cutters use 10 × magnification. The Mantis scope is a stereo-optical viewer with no eyepiece. Even though the optics are mediocre, it has the big advantage of a wide screen through which the cutters can see the work that is being performed with their head facing forward and without having to bend their neck.

Slivering Dissection

The initial step of slivering the donor tissue into smaller units is the most critical and technically exacting step. Normally, the most experienced and skilled technician will perform this task. The donor strip is fixed to a tongue depressor with a needle and the technician begins to create slivers or slices from the strip (Fig. 4.11). Instead of tongue blades, some surgeons prefer to use other cutting surfaces such as plastic sheets, and soft silicon pads.

The slivering technique has been compared to "slicing a loaf of bread", an analogy in which the loaf is the strip and the emerging slices are the slivers. The ideal sliver should have a width of one FU so that the other technicians can dissect each sliver easily. Number 10 surgical blades or razorblades encased in a razorblade holder and a jeweler's forceps are the basic instruments needed for dissection of the donor strip. All slivers are immersed in the holding solution and the other technicians start dissecting the FU grafts from the sliver (Fig. 4.12).

Follicular Unit Graft Dissection

The sliver is placed on a tongue blade or special cutting board and the technician should identify and dissect under the microscope the FUs (seen as hair follicle groupings), which mostly contain two to three hairs. Grafts are separated and counted in one, two, and three to four hair FUs.

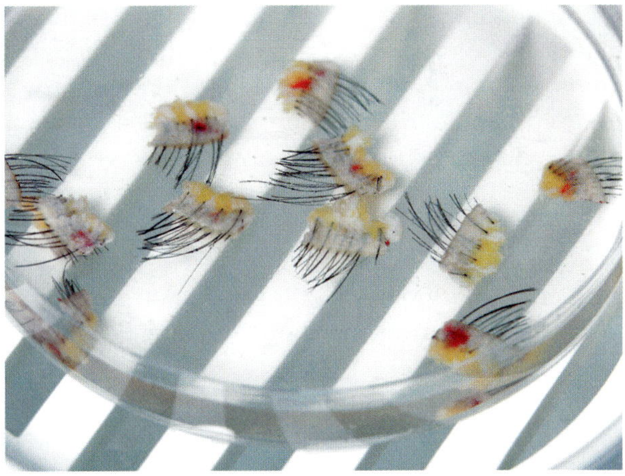

Fig. 4.12: The slivers are immediately immersed in the holding solution.

As the grafts are dissected they are immediately placed in petri dishes containing the holding solution to keep them hydrated and avoid desiccation. Some clinics prefer to have the grafts immersed completely in the holding solution, while others prefer to have the grafts on a piece of gauze in a petri dish filled with holding solution (Fig. 4.13). The first method ensures the grafts are always hydrated. The second method allows the grafts to be clustered together in order to facilitate counting, but the techs need to pay close attention to prevent desiccation. The author prefers complete immersion of the grafts in the holding solution.

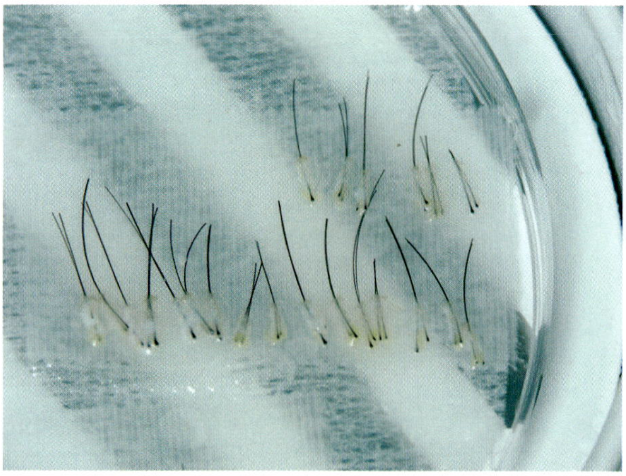

Fig. 4.13: Follicular unit grafts dissected from the slivers.

The graft cutting procedure should be performed with great care so as to obtain hair follicles with their dermal papillae and sheaths intact. Grafts should neither be too "skinny" nor too "chubby". "Skinny" grafts are more difficult to handle, and more prone to desiccation and trauma at implantation that can reduce graft survival. Excessively "chubby" grafts can also make implantation more difficult and force the surgeon to make bigger recipient sites. The perfect graft should have a pear-shape or tear-drop shape with little epidermis and little but sufficient amount of protective dermis and subcutaneous fat around the dermal papilla.

The number of cutters needed for the process of strip graft dissection in a hair transplant session varies in different practices according to the size of the session. I would recommend having at least one cutter for each 500 grafts. For example, if the plan is to perform 2,000 grafts, I would recommend four cutters, one acting initially as the sliverer and then as a cutter once slivering is finished.

Follicular Unit Extraction

In the technique of FUE, the FU is sectioned in situ, so the step of microscopic slivering and graft dissection is not needed. This is in theory a theoretical advantage provided that the hair transplant surgeon has sufficient skill and experience to harvest the majority of the FUs intact with a low rate of complete transection. In less experienced hair surgeons, however, the rate of transection can be so high that this theoretical advantage is offset by the poor quality of the grafts.

When one compares under the microscope FU dissected grafts (from strip) with FUE grafts, the microscopically dissected grafts usually have more surrounding tissue and are chubbier. The FUE grafts tend to have less fat tissue surrounding the inferior portion of the follicle. These small changes in FU histomorphology between FUE and microscopically dissected grafts should not affect hair graft survival, provided that the critical elements of the FU, the bulge stem cell region, and the dermal papillae are kept and implanted intact. The survival rate of a hair graft depends on many factors,[11] and in the author's experience, the most critical step is the trauma and manipulation of grafts at placement. In this regard, it is important to note that FUE grafts are more delicate to handle and more prone to damage during placement.

REFERENCES

1. Cole J. Aid to Hairline Design (AHD). Hair Transplant Forum Int. 2008;18:173-4.
2. Ng B, Pathomvanich D, Laorwong K. Laser-assisted hairline placement. Hair Transplant Forum Int. 2008; 18:169-72.
3. Nusbaum BP, Fuentefría S. Naturally occurring female hairline patterns. Dermatol Surg. 2009;35:907-13.
4. Shapiro R. Principles of creating a natural hairline. In: Unger W, Shapiro R, Unger R, Unger M (Eds). In: Hair Transplantation, 5th edition. London: Informa Healthcare; 2011. pp. 374-82.
5. Rose PT, Parsley WM. Science of hairline design. In: Haber RS, Stough DB (Eds). Hair Transplantation. Philadelphia, PA: Elsevier Saunders; 2006. pp. 55-71.
6. Limmer BL. Micrograft survival. In: Stough DB, Haber RS (Eds). Hair Replacement: Surgical and Medical. St. Louis: Mosby; 1996. pp. 147-50.
7. Krueger N, Sadick NS. Chapter 45: New frontiers in graft-storage solutions. In: Lam SM (Ed). Hair Transplant 360. Jaypee Brother Medical Publishers. pp. 575-82.
8. Uebel C, da Silva JB, Cantarelli D, et al. The role of platelet plasma growth factors in male pattern baldness. Plast Reconstr Surg. 2006;118:1458-66.
9. Mathew AJ. A review of cellular biopreservation considerations during hair transplantation. Hair Transplant Forum Intl. 2013;23(1):1-11.
10. Cooley JE. Bio-enhanced hair restoration. Hair Transplant Forum Intl. 2014;24(4):121-30.
11. Parsley WM, Perez-Meza D. Review of factors affecting the growth and survival of follicular grafts. J Cutan Aesthet Surg. 2010;3:69-75.

CHAPTER 5

Anesthesia and Instrumentation

Shannon Watkins

Hair transplantation is typically performed under local anesthesia. There are different tools and techniques used in hair transplant surgery. In this chapter, we discuss the various different anesthetics and instruments utilized in hair transplant surgery.

SYSTEMIC ANESTHETICS AND GENERAL CONSIDERATIONS

In our practice, we give a mild sedative such as diazepam (Valium) 5–10 mg PO prior to the procedure. Most people find it difficult to sit still for long period of time without a mild sedative. Some patients, however, prefer to and are able to undergo the procedure without sedative medications. Other hair transplant surgeons prefer to utilize conscious sedation for the hair transplant surgeries with mediations such as midazolam (benzodiazepine) with or without narcotics such as fentanyl. Short-acting medications are preferred for conscious sedation as medications must be titrated while monitoring the patient's level of arousal, respiration, oxygen saturation, pulse, blood pressure, and electrocardiography. In the United States, an anesthesiologist or certified nurse anesthesiologist should be present throughout procedures performed with conscious sedation.[1]

In our practice, we require medical clearance prior to the hair transplant surgery for patients aged 55 years or older and for those with pre-existing conditions such as diabetes. For patients on anticoagulants that cannot be discontinued for medical reasons, we do not perform the surgery due to the increased risk of bleeding complications.

ANESTHESIA FOR HAIR TRANSPLANTATION

Effective local anesthesia can be maintained for the duration of the hair transplant surgery. We accomplish this via a combination of local anesthesia and local ring blocks. Some hair transplant surgeons also incorporate nerve blocks. The cumulative dosage of local anesthetic should be monitored and there should be constant surveillance for signs of toxicity. The early signs of local anesthetic toxicity should be well known to the hair transplant surgeon, and early intervention should be executed in the unlikely event that these signs occur.[1] The signs of local anesthetic toxicity and interventions are discussed later in this chapter and are listed in Table 5.1.

History of Local Anesthesia

The ancient Incas utilized local anesthesia by chewing coca leaves and letting their saliva drip into wounds.[1,2] Local anesthesia was introduced to modern medicine by Karl Koller in 1884.[1,3] He used cocaine extracted from coca leaves as a topical anesthetic for glaucoma surgery. In 1884, Halstead performed the first regional nerve block using cocaine. In 1904, procaine was the first local anesthetic to become widely used. Lidocaine, the first "amide" local anesthetic was discovered in 1943 and remains the most popular local anesthetic to date.[1]

Table 5.1: Management of selected adverse reactions related to local anesthesia in hair transplantation.

Presenting symptoms	*Possible causes*	*Management*
Dizziness, pallor, nausea, hypotension, bradycardia	Vasovagal episode	Trendelenburg position, supportive treatment, atropine if severe/prolonged
Paresthesia of hands and feet, anxiety, dyspnea	Hyperventilation (should be apparent)	Rebreathing mask (or paper bag)
Perioral anesthesia, auditory, visual, taste disturbances	Early local anesthetic toxicity	Suspend local anesthetics, benzodiazepine IV, O_2
Convulsions	Severe anesthetic toxicity	O_2, benzodiazepines IV, intubate, hyperventilate
Decreased consciousness, hypoventilation	Benzodiazepine toxicity	O_2, flumazenil IV, consider intubation, and ventilation
Hypotension and tachycardia	Allergic reactions, check for other signs Narcotic toxicity Benzodiazepine toxicity	O_2, subcutaneous epinephrine, fluids IV, Benadryl IV, Solu-Medrol IV, ranitidine IV O_2, naloxone IV, fluids IV O_2, flumazenil IV, fluids IV
Hypotension and bradycardia	Vasovagal episode Severe local anesthetic toxicity	Trendelenburg position, supportive treatment, atropine if severe/prolonged O_2, Trendelenburg position, fluids IV, support ABCs, transfer
Hypertension and tachycardia	Vasoconstrictor reaction	O_2, metoprolol or labetalol IV if severe/prolonged, nitrates if coronary ischemia
Hypertension and bradycardia	Epinephrine and b-blocker reaction	Hydralazine or chlorpromazine IV

(IV: Intravenous).
Source: Adapted from Seager DJ, Simmons C. Local anesthesia in hair transplantation. Dermatol Surg. 2002;28(4):320-28.

Local Anesthetic Agents

"Caine" Anesthetics

These are the most popular and most effective agents used for local anesthesia. They work via blocking sodium channels on nerves, thereby blocking the conduction of nerve impulses. The "caine" anesthetics consist of a lipophilic aromatic ring connected to an intermediate chain, which is connected to a hydrophilic, ionizable amine group. The "caine" anesthetics can be divided into two groups, esters and amides, based on the intermediate linkage between the terminal amine and the aromatic ring (Fig. 5.1). Common ester anesthetics are cocaine, procaine, and tetracaine. Common amide anesthetics are lidocaine, bupivacaine, prilocaine, etidocaine, mepivacaine, and ropivacaine. The amide group, namely lidocaine and bupivacaine, are the agents most commonly used in hair transplant surgery. Liver disease, congestive heart failure, renal disease, and certain medications can limit the maximum dose allowed. There are very rare allergies to amide anesthetics, and <1% of adverse reactions reported are truly allergic.[1] The ester group is rarely used in hair transplant surgery due to a higher risk of hypersensitivity, less intense analgesia, and a shorter duration of effect.[1] The two pharmacologic classes have no cross-reactivity, so amide anesthetics can be safely given to patients with an ester anesthetic allergy.[4]

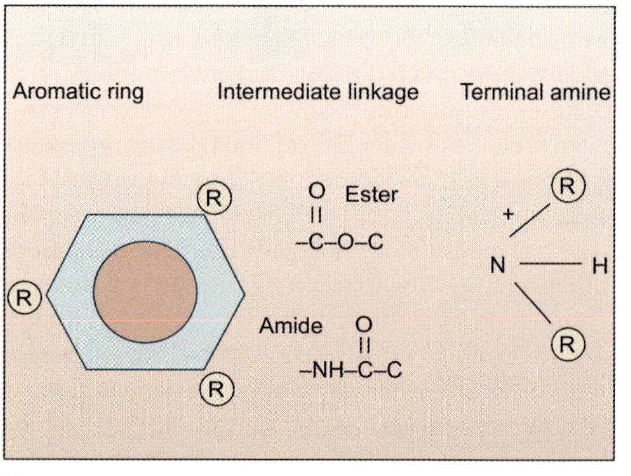

Fig. 5.1: Local anesthetic structure. Ester versus amide determined by intermediate linkage.
Source: Becker DE, Reed KL. Essentials of local anesthetic pharmacology. Anesthesia Prog. 2006;53(3):98-108; quiz 9-10.

Lidocaine Versus Bupivacaine

Lidocaine is the most commonly used local anesthetic. Some hair transplant surgeons, however, prefer bupivacaine due to its longer duration of action. Some studies have reported that plain bupivacaine lasted four to eight times longer than plain lidocaine.[1,5,6] However, one study showed that bupivacaine with epinephrine lasted only 27% longer than lidocaine with epinephrine.[1,7] Lidocaine without epinephrine lasts about 60 minutes, and lidocaine with epinephrine lasts 120 minutes. Bupivacaine without epinephrine lasts 120–240 minutes, and bupivacaine with epinephrine lasts 180–240 minutes.[4] Bupivacaine 0.25% provides similar analgesia to 1% lidocaine, as bupivacaine is four times as potent as lidocaine by weight.[1]

One advantage of lidocaine over bupivacaine is that it has a faster time to onset of anesthesia. One study reported that complete digital ring block of anesthesia was achieved in 5.8 minutes on average with lidocaine versus 11.2 minutes with bupivacaine.[1,8] With infiltration anesthesia, the onset of anesthesia can be immediate, but bupivacaine causes more infiltration pain than lidocaine.[1,7] While bupivacaine is widely and safely used by many hair transplant surgeons, one potential disadvantage of bupivacaine is that at high doses or if inadvertently injected intravascularly, it can be arrhythmogenic and can precipitate ventricular tachycardia or fibrillation that can be resistant to treatment.[1] This is not typically an issue with responsible use, so long as care is taken to avoid intravascular injection and toxic dosages are not reached. Bupivacaine rapidly blocks sodium channels and is slow to unblock them, resulting in a prolonged refractory period in cardiac tissue, which can set up re-entrant arrhythmias when intravascularly injected or at toxic doses. Bupivacaine may also affect calcium and potassium channels.[1]

Non-"caine" Anesthetic Agents and Vasoconstrictors

At present the non-"caine" anesthetics such as diphenhydramine 1%, benzyl alcohol 0.9%, and intradermal metoclopramide and tramadol do not have a role in hair transplant surgery, as they lack suitable efficacy and duration.[1]

Vasoconstrictors when added to local anesthetics can prolong the duration of anesthesia. Epinephrine is the most commonly used vasoconstrictor in North America. It has been shown to prolong the duration of local anesthesia in a dose-related fashion.[9] Vasoconstrictors limit the rate of absorption of local anesthetics and thus reduce toxicity and allow higher dosages to be used. They also facilitate hemostasis.[1] Large volumes of epinephrine injected subcutaneously or intravascularly can lead to systemic cardiovascular toxicity with increased heart rate and blood pressure. Therefore, caution should be employed to avoid intravascular injection, and also in patients with hypertension or coronary artery disease.[1]

Of note, when epinephrine is mixed with local anesthetics, it causes oxidation of lidocaine and results in 10% loss of potency per day. Sodium metabisulfite or bisulfate is added to lidocaine preparations to prevent epinephrine oxidation, but this increases the acidity of the solution that increases the injection pain[7] and may lead to tachyphylaxis or increased tolerance to further local anesthesia.[1,10] For this reason, lidocaine is often buffered with 8.4% sodium bicarbonate at a volume ration of 9:1, and bupivacaine is often buffered at a volume ratio of 50:1. Some surgeons, however, avoid buffering anesthetic solutions, as there are reports of increased edema and bleeding with buffered solutions.[4]

Maximum Dosages and Toxicity

The maximum recommended dosage for lidocaine with epinephrine is 7 mg/kg. This is 0.7 mL/kg of 1% lidocaine with epinephrine. Lidocaine 1% has 10 mg of lidocaine/1 mL. For an average 70 kg man, the maximum dose of 1% lidocaine with epinephrine would be 50 mL of 1% lidocaine with epinephrine. The maximum dose of 0.25% bupivacaine with 1:100,000 epinephrine is 225 mg or 90 mL. These maximum dosages, however, do not take into account the vascularity of the area infiltrated, the rate of usage, or the number of administrations. For example, with tumescent liposuction, up to 50 mg/kg of diluted lidocaine can be safely given,[1] so further studies are needed to explore the safety of local anesthetics in hair transplant surgery. One study investigating peak serum lidocaine concentrations after Mohs micrographic surgery, which utilizes local anesthesia of the head and neck, reported that levels of serum lidocaine did not approach toxic levels after a mean of 15 mL (range 5–48 mL) of 1% lidocaine with 1:200,000 epinephrine and 1:10 (8.4%) bicarbonate. The highest peak serum lidocaine level recorded at any time point (blood was drawn over a span of up to 8 hours) in all patients was well below the toxic level and was 0.3 mg/mL.[11]

Toxicities of local anesthetic correlate with plasma levels of the drugs. The half-life of lidocaine when injected locally (with normal liver function) is 120 minutes or 2 hours.[11] Peak serum levels of lidocaine with local anesthesia injections above the level of the clavicle were reported to be at 5.8 hours according to a study by Rubin et al.[11,12] In general, as serum lidocaine levels approach 3 mg/mL, patients can begin to experience feelings of light-headedness, dizziness, and drowsiness. The threshold for objective signs of lidocaine toxicity is 5 mg/mL; at this point, patients can experience muscle fasciculations, tinnitus, paresthesias, and some describe a metallic taste.[1] If levels exceed 9 mg/mL, seizures, coma, respiratory, and cardiac arrest can occur.[11] Neurologic symptoms typically occur at levels >4.5 mg/L but have occurred at levels <3 mg/L[1,13] (Fig. 5.2). Central nervous system (CNS) toxicity can occur with plasma bupivacaine levels of 1 mg/L, so while bupivacaine is four times as potent as lidocaine for local anesthesia it is also more potent for neurologic toxicity. A sheep study showed that a dose of 31 mg/kg of lidocaine caused death, while only 3.6 mg/kg of bupivacaine caused death. Therefore, bupivacaine is four times as potent as lidocaine but nine times as lethal.[1,14] Furthermore, it is important to note that benzodiazepines (often given as mild sedation for hair transplant surgery) can mask the early warning signs of local anesthetic toxicity. This is because local anesthetics block inhibitory neural pathways before excitatory pathways. Therefore, the first neurologic symptoms of local anesthetic toxicity tend to be excitatory (dizziness, light-headedness, visual, auditory, and taste disturbances). Since benzodiazepines are CNS depressants, they can mask the early excitatory signs of toxicity. Benzodiazepines are also a treatment for local anesthetic toxicity and should be given intravenous with oxygen if systems of local anesthetic toxicity manifest (such as perioral paresthesia, visual or auditory disturbances, and seizures). With prolonged seizures, intubation should be performed for airway protection.[1]

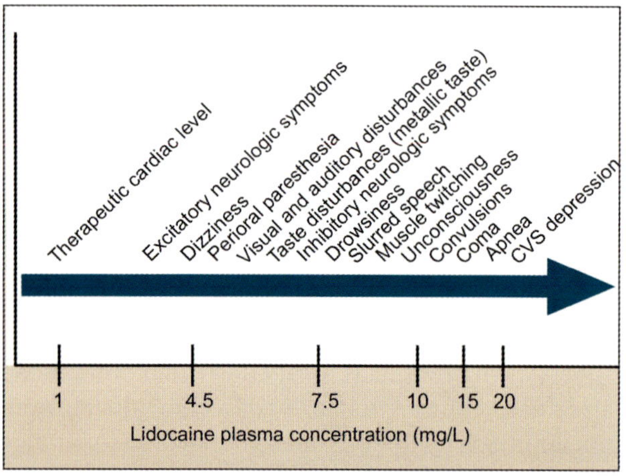

Fig. 5.2: Signs of lidocaine toxicity with escalating doses of lidocaine. *Sources*: Seager DJ, Simmons C. Local anesthesia in hair transplantation. Dermatol Surg. 2002;28(4):320-28. Bradley R Wolf. Anesthesia. In Walter Unger, Ronald Shapiro, Mark Unger, Robin Unger (Eds), Hair transplantation, 5th edition (pp. 226-246). New York: Informa Healthcare; 2011.

Prevention and Treatment of Toxicity

It is easier to prevent toxicity than to treat it. A flow sheet recording the timing and amount of local anesthesia administered as well as the cumulative dose should be kept. Proper injection technique should avoid intravascular infiltration of local anesthetic. One should continuously monitor patients for any signs of neurologic, cardiovascular, or hemodynamic instability. *See* Table 5.1 for a summary of management of selected side effects and toxicities from local anesthesia.[1] Medications such as flumazenil (antidote for valium toxicity) and naloxone (antidote for opiate toxicity) should be readily available in case of an overdose.[4]

Medication-Related Interactions

The hair transplant surgeon should be aware of potential interactions between the patient's medications and anesthetics utilized during the hair transplant surgery. Programs such as Epocrates (www.epocrates.com) can be utilized to check for medication interactions. Examples of potential interactions include antidepressants such as monoamine oxidase inhibitors and tricyclic antidepressants, which can interact with epinephrine and cause a hypertensive crisis. Dilantin and lidocaine can potentiate each other's effects as well as lead to an increased risk of methemoglobinemia. Nonspecific β-blockers (such as Inderal) can interact with epinephrine potentially, increasing the risk of hypertensive crisis, and also can interact with lidocaine, increasing plasma levels of lidocaine. These are just a few specific examples of potential drug interactions and additional interactions exist, so a thorough medication history should be taken and medications should be checked for interactions in programs such as epocrates.com to avoid unwanted complications and interactions.[4]

Techniques to Achieve Local Anesthesia in Hair Transplant Surgery

Innervation of the scalp is from branches of the supraorbital, supratrochlear, zygomaticotemporal, auriculotemporal, lesser occipital, greater occipital, and third occipital nerves (Figs. 5.3A and B).[1] To anesthetize the donor area, most practitioners use a local ring block followed by local dermal infiltration of anesthesia into the donor area. To anesthetize the recipient area, practitioners typically perform either a ring block or a combination of ring blocks with local dermal infiltration and/or a supraorbital and supratrochlear nerve blocks. Dr Swinehart in a "Letter to the Editor" describes an additional technique for recipient site anesthesia in area prone to bleeding. He empties a 30 cc bottle of 1% lidocaine with epinephrine into a petri dish with gauze sponges. Prior to insertion of recipient grafts, he recommends rubbing an anesthetic-containing sponge over the area to be transplanted. In doing so, local anesthesia soaks down into recipient "slits", further anesthetizing the area and the epinephrine further constricts vessels without any additional injections.[15]

Typical setup of local anesthetics for hair transplant surgery illustrates our typical tray of local anesthetics for hair transplant surgeries. This tray consists of four 3 cc syringes of 0.5% lidocaine + 1:100,000 epinephrine buffered with sodium bicarbonate, three 3 cc syringes of 1% lidocaine + 1:100,000 epinephrine buffered with sodium bicarbonate, three 3 cc syringes of 2% lidocaine + 1:100,000 epinephrine buffered with sodium bicarbonate, two 3 cc syringes of 0.025% Marcaine + 1:100,000 epinephrine, and three 5 cc syringes of normal saline (Fig. 5.4).

Ring Block of Scalp

A ring block involves blocking of all nerves, innervating an area by infiltrating a continuous path along the edge of the area. The needle is inserted into the subcutaneous plane and the local anesthetic solution is injected. In doing so a "ring" of anesthesia is accomplished, which can be subsequently re-enforced as necessary by intradermal injections into the target area (Fig. 5.5.). A vibration anesthesia device (Blaine Labs, Santa Fe Springs, CA) can be used to further mitigate the pain of injection. This is because concomitant physical stimulation can diminish the perception of painful stimuli.[4]

Supraorbital and Supratrochlear Nerve Blocks

A supraorbital nerve block can be performed by palpating the supraorbital notch, which lies in a vertical line drawn through the midpoint of the pupil or just medial to that line, and injecting 0.25% bupivacaine with or without 1:100,000 epinephrine, or 1% lidocaine with or without 1:100,000 epinephrine, above or below the notch with a 30-gauge needle. Approximately 1.5–2 mL of anesthetic is typically injected very slowly. It is important to ensure that the needle is outside the supraorbital foramen to avoid

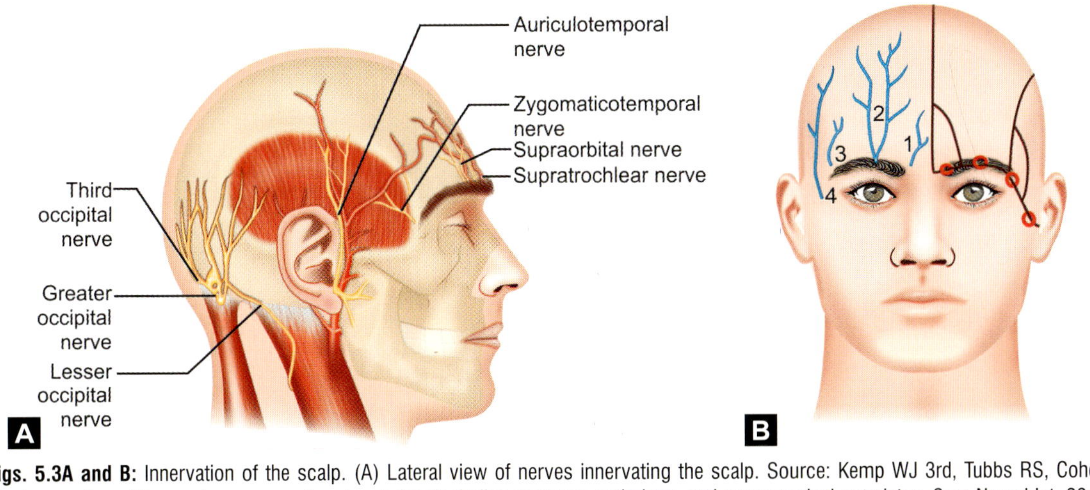

Figs. 5.3A and B: Innervation of the scalp. (A) Lateral view of nerves innervating the scalp. Source: Kemp WJ 3rd, Tubbs RS, Cohen-Gadol AA. The innervation of the scalp: a comprehensive review including anatomy, pathology, and neurosurgical correlates. Surg Neurol Int. 2011;2:178. (B) Anterior view of branches innervating the scalp including the supratrochlear, supraorbital, and zygomaticotemporal, and auriculotemporal nerves. Source: Kerscher C, Zimmermann M, Graf BM, et al. Scalp blocks. A useful technique for neurosurgery, dermatology, plastic surgery and pain therapy. Anaesthesist. 2009;58(9):949-58; quiz 959-60.

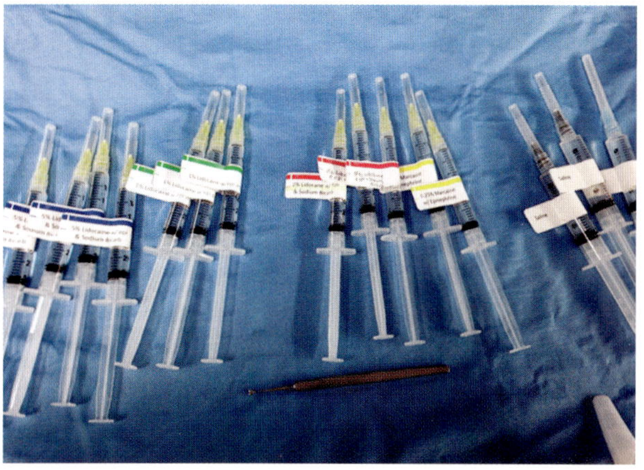

Fig. 5.4: Typical setup of local anesthetics for hair transplant surgery. From left to right: 4 × 3 cc syringes of 0.5% lidocaine + 1:100,000 epinephrine + sodium bicarbonate 3 × 3 cc syringes of 1% lidocaine + 1:100,000 epinephrine + sodium bicarbonate, 3 × 3 cc syringes of 2% lidocaine + 1:100,000 epinephrine + sodium bicarbonate, 2 × 3 cc syringes of 0.025% Marcaine + 1:100,000 epinephrine, 3 × 5 cc syringes of normal saline.

nerve damage. It is also essential to withdraw the syringe prior to injection of the anesthetic to protect against intra-arterial injection. Possible complications of nerve blocks include laceration of nerves and vessels, intravascular infiltration, ecchymosis, and temporary ptosis. A supratrochlear nerve block can be performed by injecting local anesthetic at the supraorbital rim approximately 1 cm medial to the supraorbital notch (Fig. 5.6). These nerve blocks can provide effective, durable, and comfortable anesthesia to the frontal-medial forehead and scalp.[1,16,17]

Other Techniques to Minimize the Pain of Local Anesthesia

A vibration anesthesia device can be used to further mitigate the pain (Fig. 5.7). Stimulating the touch fibers can minimize the nerves conduction of painful stimuli. This is based on the Gate Control Theory, which holds that ascending transmission of painful stimuli by slowly conducting A-delta, and C-nerve fibers can be modified by the afferent sensory stimuli of touch, pressure, and vibration, which are carried by rapidly conducing A-alpha and A-beta nerve fibers. Pain pathways can be viewed as analogous to a highway, which only so many "vehicles" or sensory stimuli can travel on at once.[4] Warming the anesthetic solution to a temperature of 37°C using dry heat or warm water baths can also reduce injection pain. A small needle caliber also minimizes pain from local anesthetic injection, so whenever possible surgeons

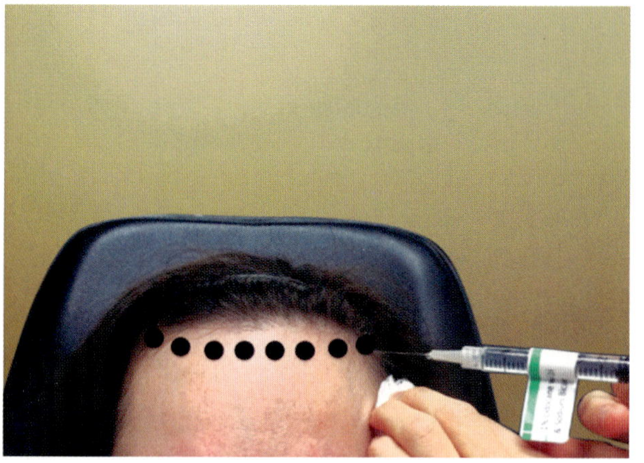

Fig. 5.5: Ring block. A ring block involves blocking of all nerves innervating an area by infiltrating a continuous path in the subcutaneous plane along the edge of the area.

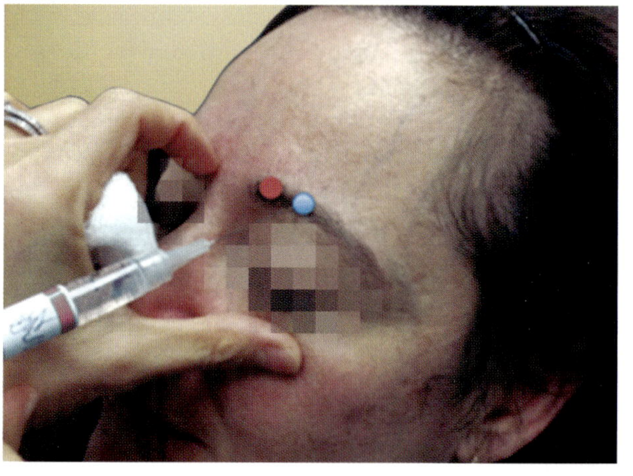

Fig. 5.6: Supraorbital nerve (blue circle) and supratrochlear nerve block (red circle). Supraorbital nerve block: palpate supraorbital notch directly above pupil. Inject vertical or slightly upward to bone. Make sure needle outside supraorbital foramen to avoid nerve damage. Inject 1.5–2 mL slowly. Supratrochlear nerve block: inject 1 mL of local anesthetic at the medial corner of orbit, a few millimeters lateral to apex of nose at the level of the eyebrow.
Source: Adapted from Kerscher C, Zimmermann M, Graf BM, Hansen E. Scalp blocks. A useful technique for neurosurgery, dermatology, plastic surgery and pain therapy. Anesthesist. 2009;58(9):949-58; quiz 959-60.

should use 30-gauge needles. Decreasing the rate of injection can also minimize pain; this can be accomplished by using larger 3-mL syringes to minimize the hydrostatic pressure and rate of injection of local anesthetic.[4]

INSTRUMENTATION FOR HAIR TRANSPLANT SURGERY

Patient comfort is critical given the relatively long duration of hair transplant surgery. Many hair transplant

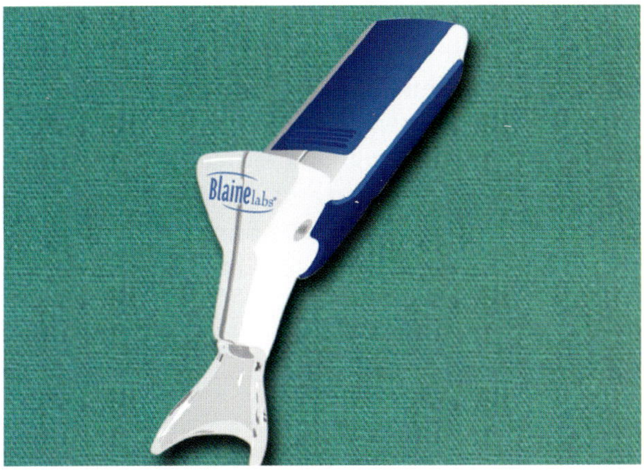

Fig. 5.7: Vibration anesthesia device by Blaine Labs.
Source: http://blainelabs.com/product/pain-management/vibration-anesthesia-device/

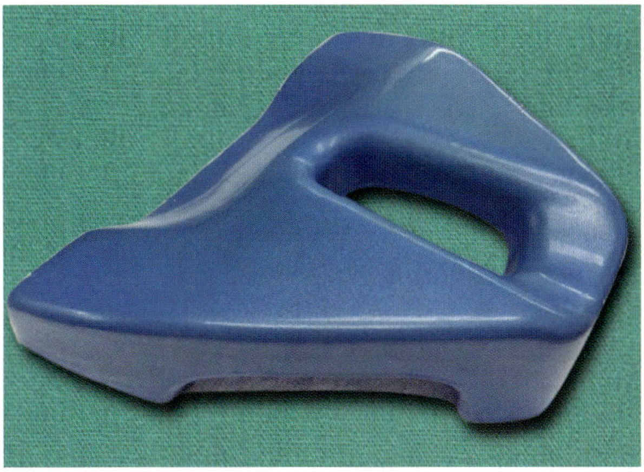

Fig. 5.8: Specialized pillow for head support during donor harvesting (Pron-Pillo).

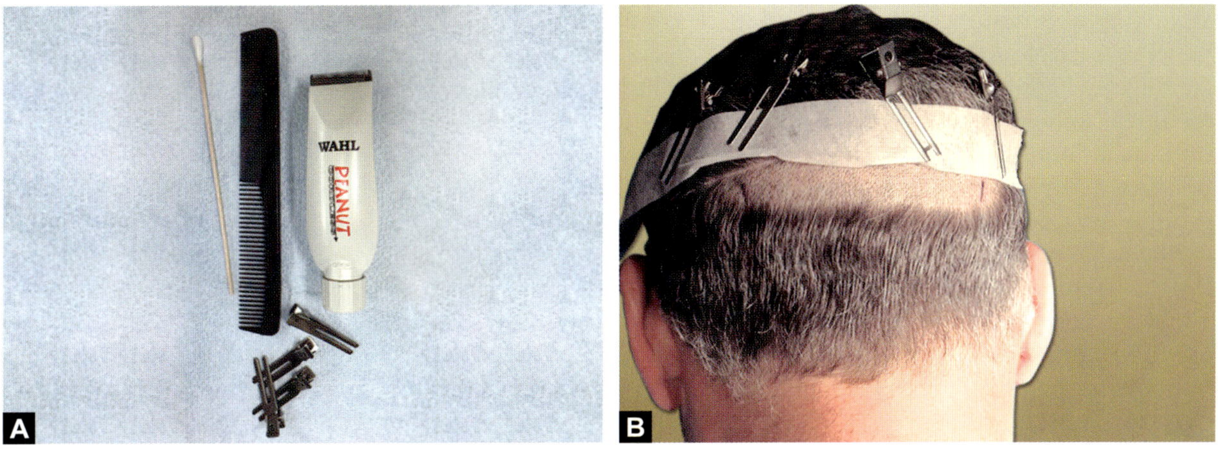

Figs. 5.9A and B: Preparation of donor area. (A) Tools utilized to prepare donor area for harvesting: wooden Q-tip, fine-tooth comb, Wahl peanut mustache trimmer, and stainless steel hair clips. (B) Patient prepped for donor harvesting.

surgeons utilize a specially designed pillow with room for the face to maximize patient comfort while patients are in the prone position for donor harvesting. The patient may need to be in the prone position for a prolonged time, especially with follicular unit extraction (FUE) (Fig. 5.8). Many also utilize a small standard pillow for head support during the transplantation of the recipient area.

Donor Harvesting Instruments

Instruments for Donor Ellipse Harvesting/Strip Harvesting

Donor harvesting is typically performed using a No. 10 or 15 Personna blade, with either a single- or double-blade approach. Prior to donor harvesting, a mustache trimmer, comb, paper tape, and hair clips are utilized to prepare the donor area for harvesting (Figs. 5.9A and B). Standard forceps and skin hooks can be used to retract the scalp skin and directly visual hair follicles, thereby minimizing follicle transection. A standard needle driver, forceps, and 3.0 sutures [nylon, Prolene, or polydioxanone suture (PDS)], or forceps and a staple gun are utilized to close the scalp defect (Fig. 5.10).

Instruments for FUE

The pros and cons of the various different methods for FUE are discussed in detail in Chapter 3. Here, we briefly review the most commonly used instruments for FUE.

Manual FUE Devices

Follicular unit extraction is the method by which individual follicular units are extracted from the donor

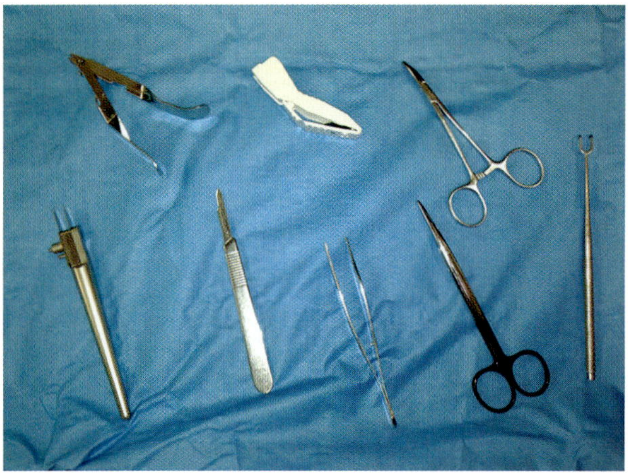

Fig. 5.10: Standard instruments for elliptical excision of donor hair. Top row: 3M Skin Staple Remover, 3M Precise MS Skin Stapler, Kelly Clamp. Bottom row: double-bladed scalpel, single-bladed scalpel, skin forceps, tissue cutting scissors, and skin hook (note usually two skin hooks are in setup).

area. This technique uses small circular trephine punches to isolate and extract follicular units. Follicular unit extraction offers the advantage of eliminating the linear donor scar of traditional ellipse harvesting. This is important to many patents who want to preserve the option to wear shorter hair styles in the future.

There are many factors to consider when purchasing an FUE device. Different punches may vary in metal type, punch edge sharpness, punch diameter, cutting edge location, punch wall thickness, and punch edge shape (smooth versus contoured). Different hair transplant surgeons have different preferences with regard to these various different qualities.

There are three important diameters with respect to an FUE punch: (1) internal diameter (distance between internal margins of the punch), (2) external diameter (distance between outer margins of the punch), and (3) cutting diameter (distance between the cutting edges of the punch). There are three cutting edge styles as well: (1) inside margin cutting edge with outside bevel (type 5 punch), (2) middle margin cutting edge with a middle bevel (type 4 punch), and (3) outside margin cutting edge with an inside bevel (type 3 punch). Some authors feel that the outside margin cutting edge with inside bevel (type 3 punch) improves tissue cutting, reduces follicle trauma, and is best for high-quality extractions, but opinions vary[18] (Fig. 5.11A).

In terms of punch size variation, some hair transplant surgeons vary the size of the punches based on follicular transection rates. With higher transection rates, the size of the punch can be increased to accommodate for factors such as larger follicular groupings or those with more splaying. Punch diameter sizes used in FUE typically vary from 0.75 to 1.25 mm in diameter.[18] Contoured surface punches are also available. A contoured surface punch is designed to reduce the friction and axial force required to penetrate the skin (Fig. 5.11B). Some hair transplant surgeons also use the standard 1 mm punch trephine utilized for punch biopsies (Fig. 5.11C).[18]

Motorized FUE Devices

Many different motorized FUE devices exist. They all rely on the skill and accuracy of the operator to harvest follicular units with minimal transection. Two of the more popular devices include the SAFE system (Fig. 5.12) and the Neograft system. The SAFE system is a motorized FUE device invented by James Harris. It is composed of a 1 mm sharp and a 1 mm dull punch. The 1 mm sharp punch scores the dermis around the follicular unit to a depth of 0.3–0.5 mm, while the dull punch dissects the follicular unit out to a depth of 4 mm. The average transection rate of the SAFE system reported by Harris was 6.14% (range 1.7–15%).[19] The Neograft machine is a powered handheld device that uses a sharp punch biopsy to extract follicular units from the donor area. Extracted hairs are removed by the machine via a controlled pneumatic pressure system and stored in a saline-filled canister until they are implanted in the recipient area. Multiple other motorized FUE devices exist and also depend on the operator for accuracy.

Artas Robotic FUE Device

The Artas Robotic System approved by the Food and Drug Administration for hair transplantation in 2011 is the only truly robotic system for FUE on the market (Figs. 5.13A and B). The Artas Robotic System utilizes a 1 mm punch with a "needle-within-needle" design attached to a robotic arm to harvest donor grafts. There is a sharp inner punch surrounded by a blunt outer punch. The sharp inner punch creates a shallow 1 mm incision and subsequently the blunt outer punch spinning at 400–800 rpm dissects and separates the follicular units from surrounding tissue. A suction system elevates the graft from the surrounding skin. Technicians then manually harvest the grafts. A combination of stereoscopic cameras managed by image processing software allows the robot to identify the precise angle and direction of hair growth and adjust the angle of harvest in real time to accurately harvest grafts. Because

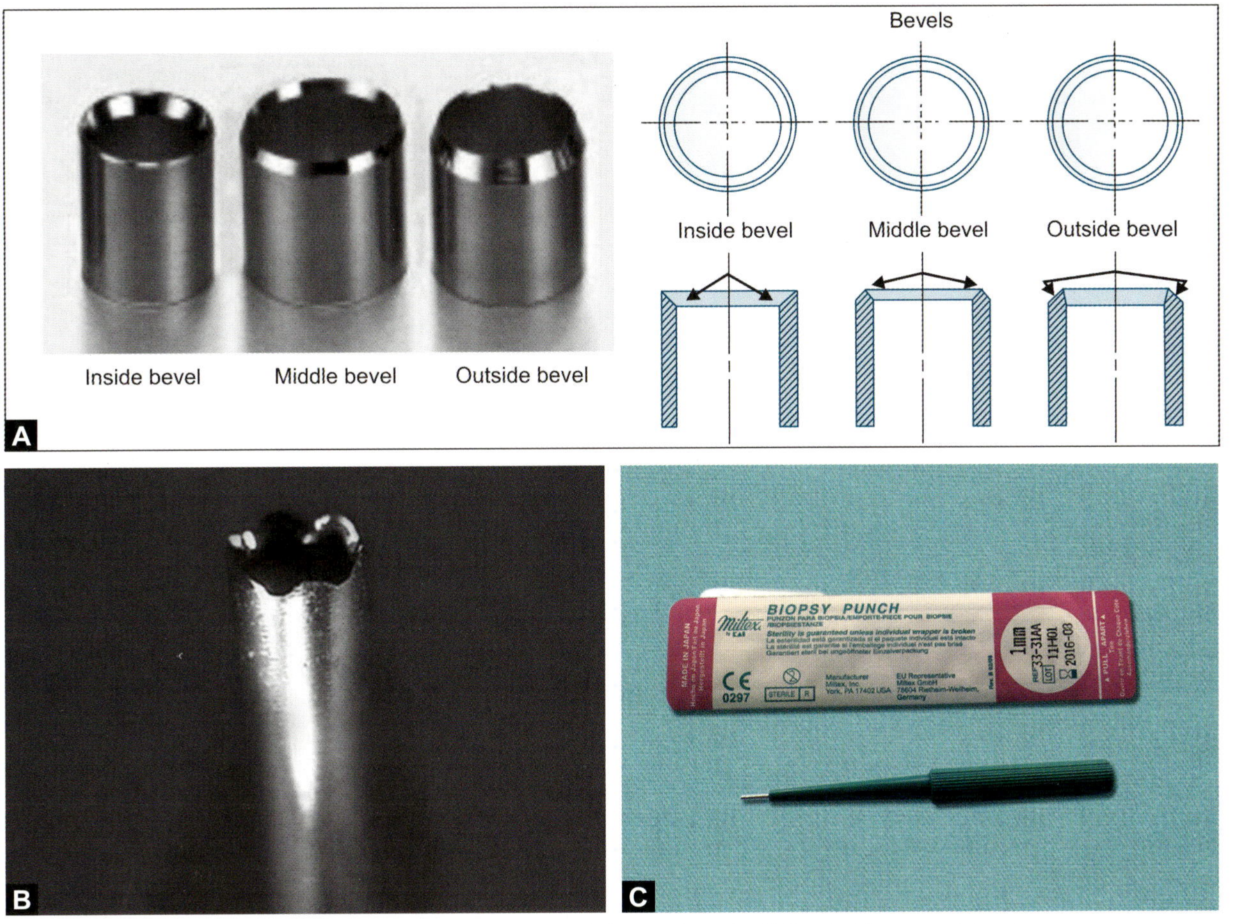

Figs. 5.11A to C: Punch edge styles. (A) Punch edge bevel location. (B) Contoured punch. (C) Standard 1 mm punch trephine.
Source: Figures 5.11A and B Reprinted from Cole JP. "An Analysis of follicular punches, mechanics, and dynamics in follicular unit extraction. Facial Plast Surg Clin North Am. 2013;21(3):437-47, with permission from Elsevier.

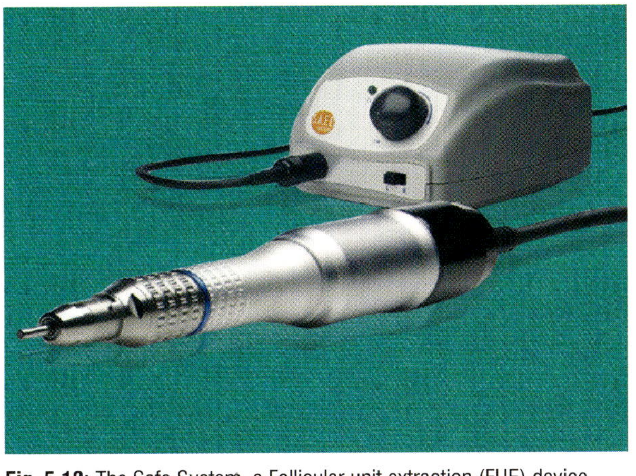

Fig. 5.12: The Safe System, a Follicular unit extraction (FUE) device.
Source: Image courtesy of Dr. James Harris. www.hsccolorado.com.

of the high level of automation, the robot is able to remove 400–600 grafts per hour.[20] Significant financial cost and space requirement has been a barrier to investment in this device for some hair transplant surgeons (Table 5.2). Figure 5.13B shows the instruments needed for donor harvesting with the Artas Robotic System.

Instruments for Graft Preparation

Forceps and straight Personna blades (Personna Medical, Verona, VA) are the standard instruments used for graft preparation (Fig. 5.14A). For Afro centric hair, which often can have a "c-shaped" curve, some hair transplant surgeons recommend using a Dermablade (Personna Medical, Verona, VA) for graft preparation that can be bent to match the shape of the curl[21]; others manually bend a straight Personna blade to match the shape of the hair (Fig. 5.14B). Some technicians prefer to utilize an LED magnifier or a microscope to increase the accuracy and precision of graft dissection (Figs. 5.15A and B).

Table 5.2: Product specifications for artas robotic system.

	Artas robotic follicular unit extraction
Time to harvest grafts	45–60 minutes for 300–600 grafts, 60–120 minutes for 600–1,200 grafts
Healing time	3–5 days
Cost	Significant to purchase machine and additional per surgery fee for each harvest attempt
Transection rate	Low to low-moderate
Physician skill	Knowledge of software program and robot
Technician skill	Skilled technician needed to remove grafts from scalp and assess quality under magnification before placing in recipient site
Reliability	Technician + physician + robot dependent
Space requirement	Minimum office space: 10 ft × 10 ft; large procedural space Robot dimensions Cart: length (*l*), 48 in.; width (*w*), 27 in.; height (*h*), 68 in. Chair: *l*, 57 in.; *w*, 33 in.; *h*, 48 in. Weight: cart, 872 lb; chair, 550 lb
Electrical requirement	208 VAC ± 10%, single phase, 50/60 Hz, 10 A. Required power outlet configuration is NEMA L6-20R twist lock
Technical requirements	Ethernet port, no WiFi Personal computer Secondary monitor, with HDMI cables from robot to monitor Desk (workstation), at least 2′ × 3′ working surface

Source: Adapted from Avram MR, Watkins SA. Robotic follicular unit extraction in hair transplantation. Dermatol Surg. 2014;40(12):1319-27.

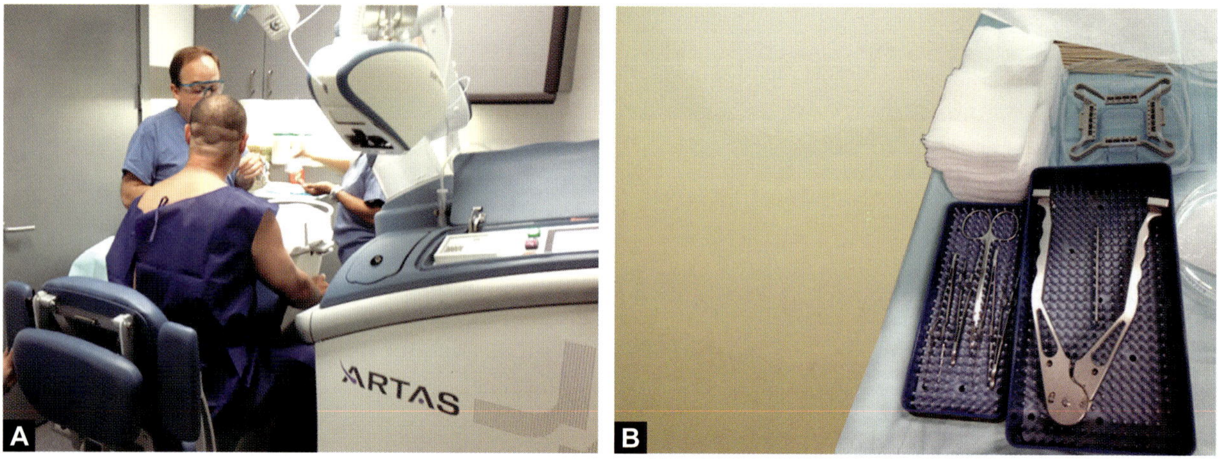

Figs. 5.13A and B: (A) Artas Robotic System. (B) Instruments utilized for harvesting with Artas Robotic System. Equipment for follicular unit extraction with Artas Robot.

Instruments for Recipient Site Creation

Recipient sites can be created with a variety of different instruments. Perhaps the most common and readily available instruments are the 18-, 19-, and 20-gauge needles. These measure 1.27 mm (18 gauge), 1.09 mm (19 gauge), and 0.9 mm (20 gauge) in diameter, respectively.[22] Needles can be bent to accommodate the length of the individual graft. Eighteen-gauge needles are typically used for three hair grafts. Nineteen-gauge needles are typically used for two hair grafts. Twenty-gauge needles are typically used for one hair grafts[16] (Fig. 5.16A). Needles utilized for recipient site creation.

Our office uses SP (spear point/spear tip) 88s (1.00 mm) and SP 89s (1.25 mm wide) attached to a lightening knife handle for recipient site creation (Fig. 5.16B). The length of the spear point tip can be adjusted to accommodate hair grafts.

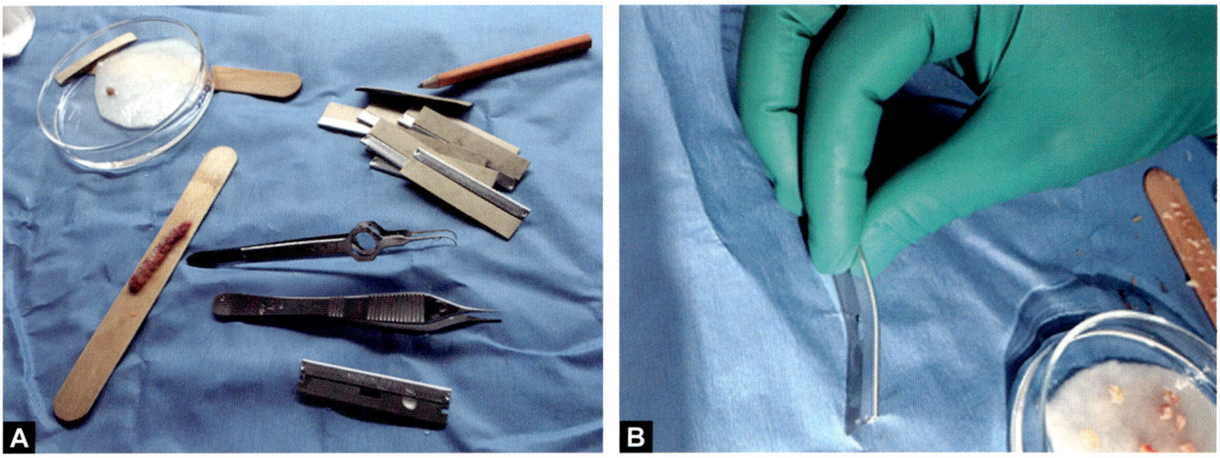

Figs. 5.14A and B: (A) Forceps and straight blades for graft preparation. (B) Personna straight blade that has been bent manually to match the curve of donor hair.

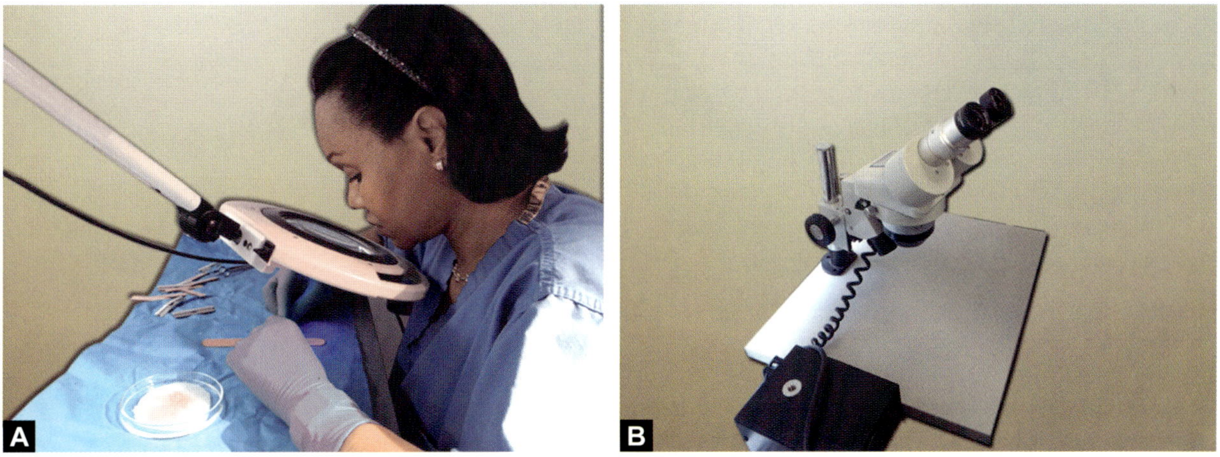

Figs. 5.15A and B: Magnifying devices utilized for creation of donor grafts. (A) LED magnifier. (B) Microscope used for dissection of donor grafts.

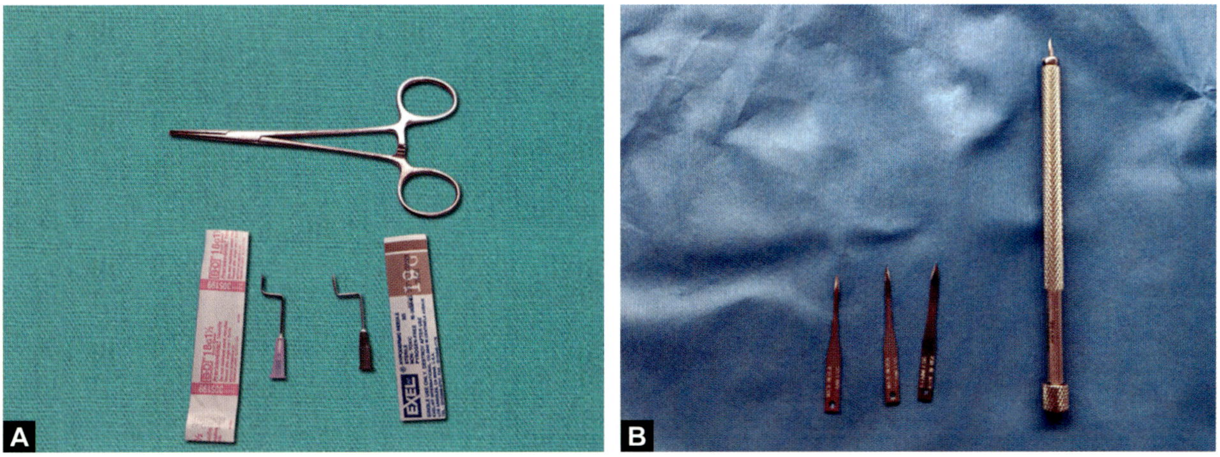

Figs. 5.16A and B: Instruments for graft site creation. (A) 18- and 19-gauge needle, and needle holder used to bend tip of needles to correct depth. (B) Spear point blades (sizes from left to right: 88, 89, 91) and lightening knife.

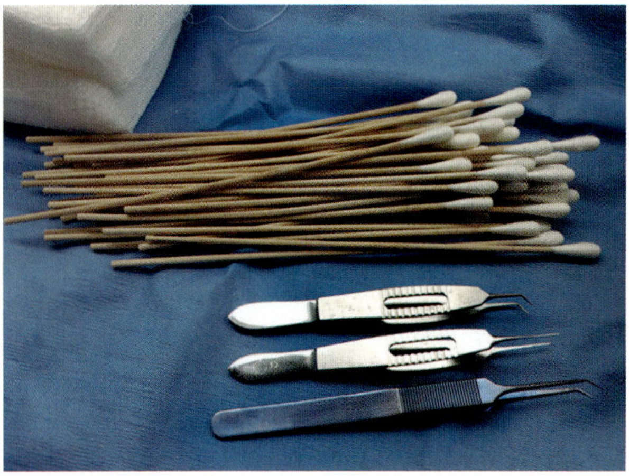

Fig. 5.17: Microvascular forceps and cotton tip applicators for graft placement.

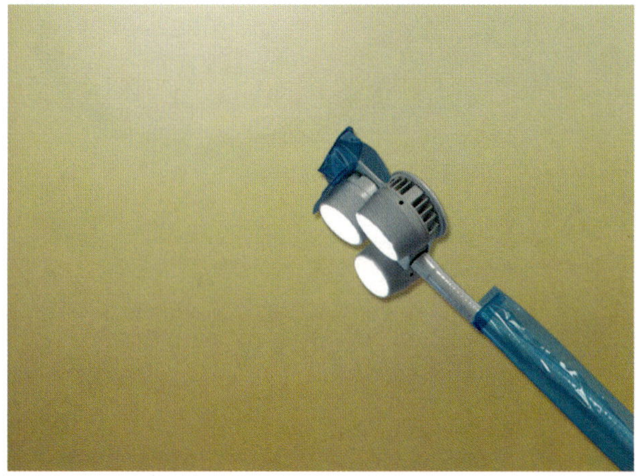

Fig. 5.18: LED light.

Some hair transplant surgeons utilize stamps to create "stamp templates" on the recipient scalp to ensure the desired recipient density is attained. Stamps of different densities can be used with either gentian violet or methylene blue to create a template on the recipient scalp. Most hair transplant surgeons, however, prefer to rely on experience and visual technique to create randomly distributed recipient sites with the desired density.

Instruments Used for Graft Placement

Specialized instruments, such as microvascular forceps with curved or straight tips, are used during graft placement (Fig. 5.17). Assistants lightly grasp perifollicular tissue above the base of the follicle to preserve the architecture of the follicle. Many assistants use a cotton-tipped applicator to help keep the graft in place and minimize bleeding and prevent "popping" of the grafts (when the grafts come out of their sites). The ideally placed graft should sit approximately 1 mm above the surrounding tissue. Grafts placed too deeply can result in pitting; those placed too superficially can result in tenting.[21]

Lighting Equipment and Ergonomics

Good lighting and ergonomics are essential in hair transplant surgery. LED lighting is helpful, as it generates less heat that translates into greater comfort for the patient (Fig. 5.18). For recipient site creation, surgeons often utilize LED surgical Loupes for magnification to allow for accurate recipient site creation with minimal injury to existing hairs (Fig. 5.19).

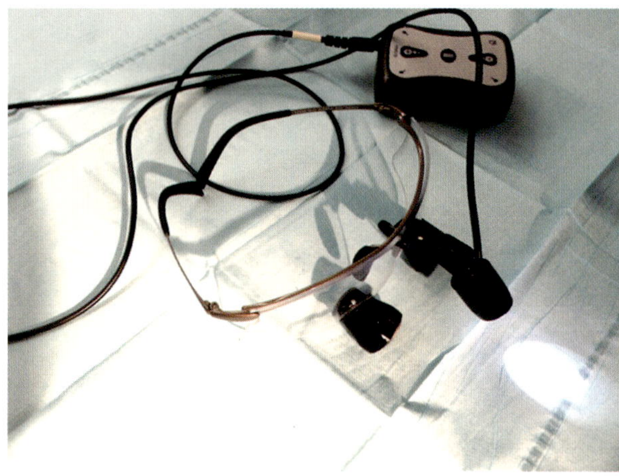

Fig. 5.19: Loops with LED light.

REFERENCES

1. Seager DJ, Simmons C. Local anesthesia in hair transplantation. Dermatol Surg. 2002;28(4):320-28.
2. Greenbaum SS, Greenbaum C. Aesthetic dermatology. In: Parish LC (Ed). McGraw-Hill; 1991.
3. Fink BR. Leaves and needles: the introduction of surgical local anesthesia. Anesthesiology. 1985;63(1):77-83.
4. Bradley R Wolf. Anesthesia. In Walter Unger, Ronald Shapiro, Mark Unger, Robin Unger (Eds), Hair transplantation, 5th edition (pp. 226-246). New York: Informa Healthcare; 2011.
5. Maimon WN, Schuller DE. Lidocaine v bupivacaine in facial plastic surgery. A clinical trial. Arch Otolaryngol. 1984;110(8):525-8.
6. Spivey WH, McNamara RM, MacKenzie RS, et al. A clinical comparison of lidocaine and bupivacaine. Ann Emer Med. 1987;16(7):752-7.

7. Howe NR, Williams JM. Pain of injection and duration of anesthesia for intradermal infiltration of lidocaine, bupivacaine, and etidocaine. J Dermatol Surg Oncol. 1994;20(7):459-64.
8. Reichl M, Quinton D. Comparison of 1% lignocaine with 0.5% bupivacaine in digital ring blocks. J Hand Surg. 1987;12(3):375-6.
9. Liu S, Carpenter RL, Chiu AA, et al. Epinephrine prolongs duration of subcutaneous infiltration of local anesthesia in a dose-related manner. Correlation with magnitude of vasoconstriction. Reg Anesth. 1995;20(5):378-84.
10. Cohen EN, Levine DA, Colliss JE, et al. The role of pH in the development of tachyphylaxis to local anesthetic agents. Anesthesiology. 1968;29(5):994-1001.
11. Alam M, Ricci D, Havey J, et al. Safety of peak serum lidocaine concentration after Mohs micrographic surgery: a prospective cohort study. J Am Acad Dermatol. 2010;63(1):87-92.
12. Rubin JP, Xie Z, Davidson C, et al. Rapid absorption of tumescent lidocaine above the clavicles: a prospective clinical study. Plast Reconstr Surg. 2005;115(6):1744-51.
13. McCaughey W. Adverse effects of local anaesthetics. Drug Safety. 1992;7(3):178-89.
14. Bacsik CJ, Swift JQ, Hargreaves KM. Toxic systemic reactions of bupivacaine and etidocaine. Oral Surg Oral Med Oral Pathol Oral Radiol Endod. 1995;79(1):18-23.
15. Swinehart JM. Local anesthesia in hair transplant surgery. Dermatol Surg. 2002;28(12):1189.
16. Lam SM. Hair transplant and local anesthetics. Clin Plast Surg. 2013;40(4):615-25.
17. Kerscher C, Zimmermann M, Graf BM, et al. Scalp blocks. A useful technique for neurosurgery, dermatology, plastic surgery and pain therapy. Anaesthesist. 2009;58(9):949-58; quiz 959-60.
18. Cole JP. An analysis of follicular punches, mechanics, and dynamics in follicular unit extraction. Facial Plast Surg Clin North Am. 2013;21(3):437-47.
19. Harris JA. New methodology and instrumentation for follicular unit extraction: lower follicle transection rates and expanded patient candidacy. Dermatol Surg. 2006;32(1):56-61; discussion 61-2.
20. Rose PT, Nusbaum B. Robotic hair restoration. Dermatol Clin. 2014;32(1):97-107.
21. Rogers NE, Callender VD. Advances and challenges in hair restoration of curly Afrocentric hair. Dermatol Clin. 2014;32(2):163-71.
22. Avram M, Rogers N. Contemporary hair transplantation. Dermatol Surg. 2009;35(11):1705-19.

CHAPTER

6

Female Hair Transplant Surgery

Robin Unger

INTRODUCTION

Hair transplant surgery for women has been growing in popularity and has become an increasingly viable treatment option for various forms of alopecia.[1] In some ways, the procedure is similar to that performed for male patients; however, there are crucial differences that need to be considered, which affect both the surgical planning and technical aspects of the procedure. One frequently debated topic is candidacy: some hair transplant surgeons maintain that only 5–10% of women are candidates for surgery, while others maintain that only a minority of women are unsuitable for surgery.[2]

This wide variance in opinions is based on the evaluation of the donor:recipient ratio from the perspective of surgeons accustomed to evaluating male patients. The vital difference is that male pattern baldness results in complete alopecia in a large area, while female pattern hair loss (FPHL) is characterized by more diffuse thinning and rarely causes complete alopecia. The goal in treating FPHL is *not* to treat all the thinning areas, but rather to increase density in the most cosmetically sensitive areas. For this reason, the author has maintained the position, for >15 years, that the majority of women can benefit from hair transplant surgery procedures.

CONSULTATION

The initial consultation is exceptionally important. The patient's medical history, family history of hair loss, and the rate of her hair loss can provide important clues about the underlying reason for the alopecia. In some cases, medical therapy can slow and potentially reverse some of the hair loss. These options need to be addressed prior to any surgical intervention.[3] The patient's age, pattern of loss, and degree of loss can also provide clues as to which medical causes may be contributing to the condition.

Dermoscopy is an invaluable tool in evaluation. It can assist in determining the degree of miniaturization in both the donor and recipient areas, which, in turn, can help predict the expected future loss. Dermoscopy can also help diagnose certain underlying conditions, including, but not limited to, alopecia areata, alopecia areata incognita, severe seborrhoea, lichen planopilaris (LPP), frontal fibrosing alopecia (FFA), folliculitis decalvans, and typical female pattern hairloss.[4,5] If there is any doubt about the underlying cause of the alopecia, one should perform two 4.0-mm biopsies and send them to a dermatopathologist with expertise in hair.

There has been an increase in diagnosed cases of LPP and FFA in this author's practice, and it is unclear as to whether this is due to the combination of dermoscopy and good dermatopathology or a true increase in incidence. Any *active* LPP or FFA disease is an absolute contraindication to surgery, and, therefore, it is very important to rule out the diagnoses prior to proceeding. If the disease has been quiescent for a minimum of 1 year, hair transplant surgery can be performed. The patient needs to be well educated on the risk of recurrence and need for lifelong surveillance.

The next aspect in the evaluation of the donor and recipient areas is to assess the density and degree of miniaturization in the donor area (Fig. 6.1). This will guide the surgeon's operative planning. On average, women in this author's practice have approximately 2,000–5,000 follicular units (FUs) available for transplantation. This limited number of available grafts makes the decision of how, where, and when to utilize them of greatest importance.

SURGICAL PLAN

Before proposing any one particular plan to the patient, it is best to ask an open-ended question: "What area do *you* think is most important?" This will help focus the conversation and clarify exactly what can be accomplished. It is better to avoid surgery if the patient's objectives are completely out of line with what can be accomplished. If the area she would

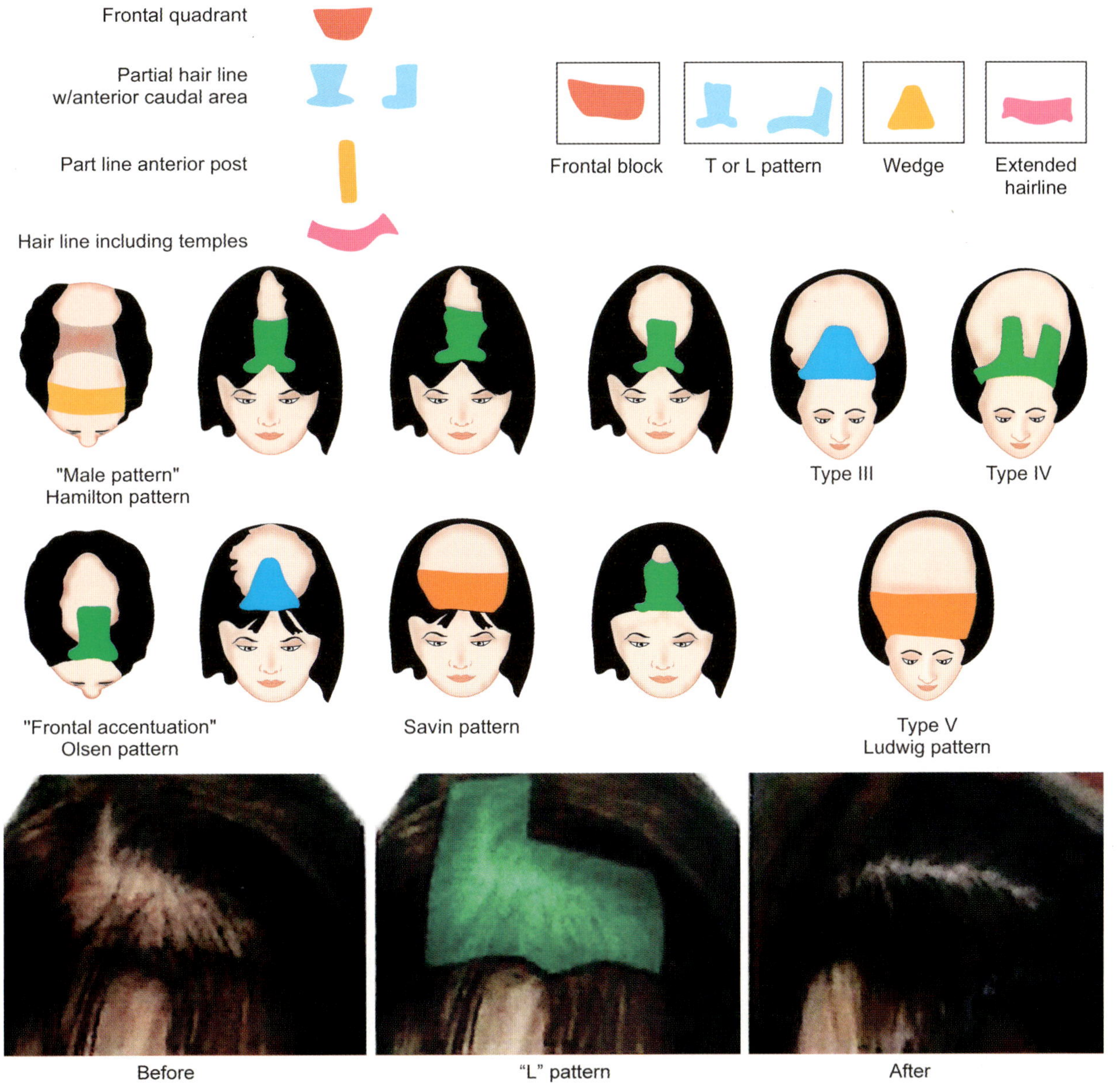

Fig. 6.1: Diagrams showing the most effective patterns for hair transplantation in women with varying degrees of hair loss. The chosen pattern depends on the amount of available donor hair, the patient's age at presentation and expected severity of loss, as well as the hairstyle that will be most complimentary and will best camouflage other thinning areas.

like to be treated is the entire caudal region and her parietal areas, then she is unlikely to be happy with what surgery can achieve and it is better to give her other options for camouflage.

The approach this author prefers is to first graft the area of greatest *long-term* cosmetic significance. Occasionally, a patient will come with a primary complaint of thinning in the vertex. It is important to caution her strongly against using the limited number of grafts in that region—as her frontal region and/or part line will definitely be more important in the future. If there is sufficient donor after the primary area of importance has been surgically treated, it may be an option to treat less important areas in the future. However, this surgeon always tries to leave some available donor hair to compensate for future loss of pre-existing hair in the cosmetically most important areas. Now, almost 15 years after starting practice, <10 patients have returned for a second surgery in the areas of primary concern.

The surgical treatment area should be chosen on the basis of the patient's natural hair directions and flow, and the hairstyle that will help achieve the greatest illusion of density. Photos can be extremely helpful in the decision-making process, allowing the patient to see the different hairstyles and areas of concern through a more powerful objective *lens.* Some patients are essentially doing a side sweep in order to provide camouflage of thinning areas—this is not the part line that would be thickened, rather it is where her natural part would occur. Together the physician and the patient (and sometimes a spouse, friend or hairstylist) can choose one or two areas that are most cosmetically important. This author described the four or five most strategic areas to treat in women. These patterns were based on years of experience and observing the impact that can be achieved with different distributions of hair.[6]

Hairline

Although hairline design is crucial with a male patterned hair loss, it is less of a priority in women. To begin with, many women have a patterned loss in which the frontal hairline is preserved. Further thickening of it can, in fact, accentuate the thinning posteriorly that is the patient's main concern. Second, many women wear their hair in such a way that the hairline is not typically visible (such as a fringe) or perhaps only visible in a small region of the part line (Figs. 6.2A and B). Nonetheless, some outline of a hairline should still be created in such cases. One can use low-density FUs in an existing strong hairline, to fortify it in case the patient has significant future loss.

Sometimes the hairline does need to be strengthened or recreated. It is best to look at previous photos of the patient in order to try to mimic the original contour. Although the transplanted one may be a little superior to the younger version. Hair transplant surgeons have proposed formulas frequently for designing the female hairline. This author has found that the variations among individuals are so extensive that the chosen hairline should actually be determined by carefully weighing the patient's current needs, available donor hair, and previous natural hairline.

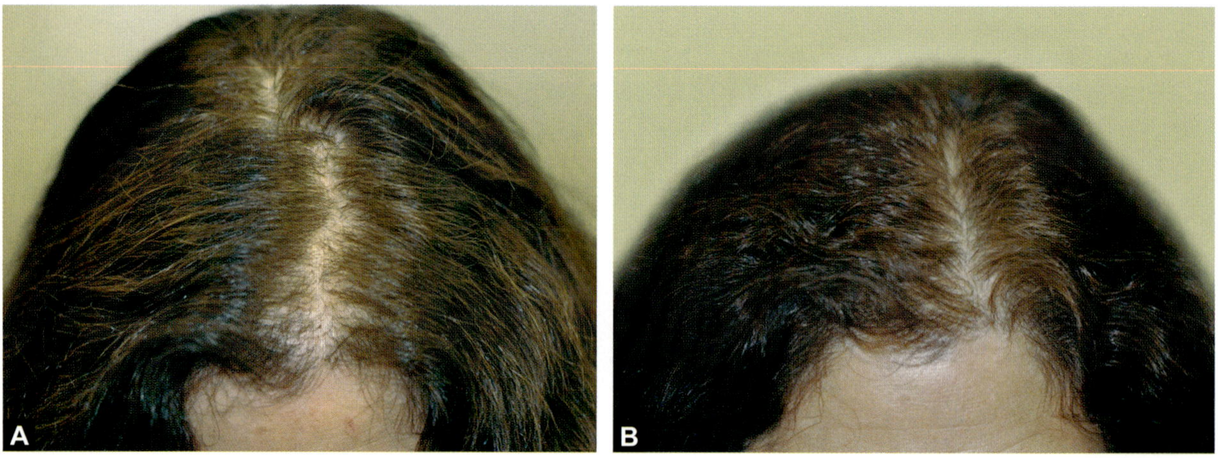

Figs. 6.2A and B: Before and after one hair transplant surgery in a female who wears her hair with a frontal or side part fringe. The hairline itself is not as aesthetically important as the frontal core. A low-density hairline (20 FU/cm^2) was created to keep the look natural even if the wind blows. The higher density frontal core area has a mixture of different size grafts and density is approximately 30 FU/cm^2.

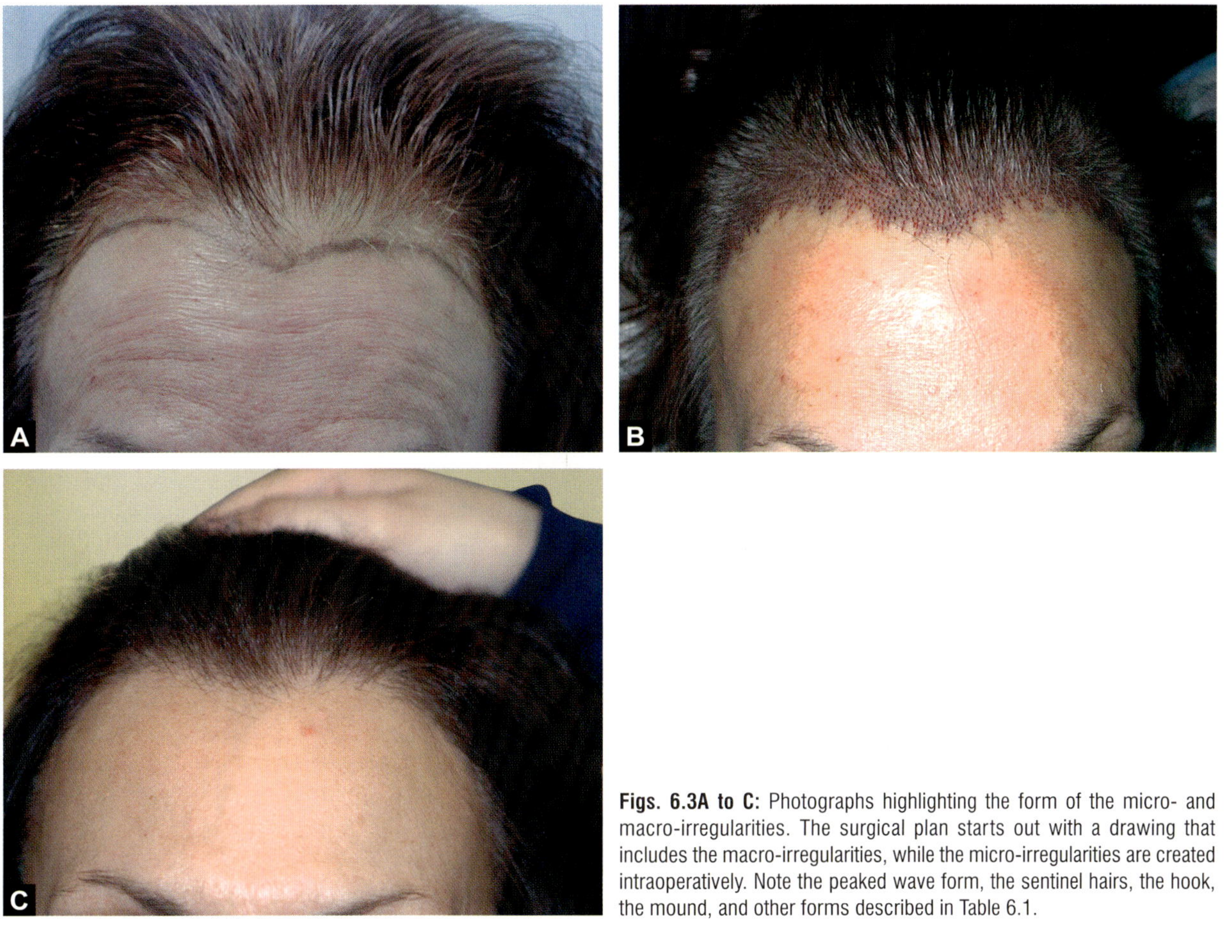

Figs. 6.3A to C: Photographs highlighting the form of the micro- and macro-irregularities. The surgical plan starts out with a drawing that includes the macro-irregularities, while the micro-irregularities are created intraoperatively. Note the peaked wave form, the sentinel hairs, the hook, the mound, and other forms described in Table 6.1.

The contour should also compliment the patient's facial features. Patients may become so focused on magazine pictures of people's hairlines that they do not consider the shape or features of their faces. Despite its name, hair transplant surgery involving the hairline is frequently *not* about the hair, it is about the frame of the face. As the superior and lateral hairline recedes, the observer's eye changes its focus; the eyes appear smaller, the nose bigger, the face broader, the temples more concave, etc. Restoring the hairline makes the patients feel as though they look more *like themselves* again.

For the past several years, this author has drawn the hairline border including the macro-irregularities. In the past, she noted that a large macro-irregularity could actually alter the overall contour of the hairline. After the initial line is created on the day of surgery, with the designated macro-irregularities, the micro-irregularities are added to create a more natural appearance (Figs. 6.3A to C). Table 6.1 shows some of the patterns that the author uses to create a natural hairline. The irregularities themselves need to be irregular and close observations of thousands of natural female hairlines revealed these naturally occurring "patterns" of irregularities.

Table 6.1: Patterns used to create a natural hairline.

Hook:	
Mound:	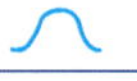
Triangle:	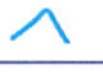
Spear:	
Sentinel hairs:	
Peaked wave:	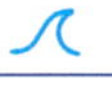
Rounded wave:	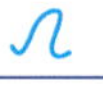

Third (and this is also true for male hair transplantation), there should be a significant *increase* in density from anterior to posterior and centrally. If the anterior hairline itself is created with a high density of hair, the posterior area needs to be treated with even higher density in order to look natural. This, in turn, results in virtually all the donor hair being utilized in a very small region of the recipient area. Therefore, even though the hairlines are a very important part of the surgical plan, they should not be created with very high densities. The author utilizes only one-haired grafts in the micro-irregularities and in the first 3–4 rows of the hairline, then progresses to two-haired grafts for 2–3 rows, and then larger ones more posteriorly (Figs. 6.4A and B).

PREOPERATIVE DIRECTIONS AND LAB TESTS

In our office, all patients are required to undergo basic preoperative lab tests. If any abnormal values of concern are noted, a full evaluation and medical clearance are required. The preoperative directions in their entirety can be seen in other texts.[7] It is important to be alert to two characteristics that are often found in women: the longer hair length and the more superficial and delicate vasculature. These features can make postoperative edema and bruising more severe and can also exaggerate the impact of any telogen effluvium postoperatively. Patients are asked to use topical minoxidil 3.5% in the surgical area starting at least 2 weeks prior to surgery, in order to potentially minimize postoperative telogen effluvium. They are also advised to limit their salt intake pre and postoperatively, and also to avoid foods, supplements, and medications that can cause excessive bleeding. The latter point is especially important in female patients because there is pre-existing hair, some of which may last their lifetime, which needs to be protected during the procedure. Excessive bleeding can make visualization and hence protection of these hairs more challenging.

Women who have been using extensions are asked to remove these if they are worn near the recipient or donor surgical areas. The author also strongly recommends that the patients follow the homeopathic regimen to help reducing bruising and forehead swelling. This includes the use of arnica tablets thrice daily and vitamin C starting 2 weeks before surgery and continuing up to 2 weeks after surgery as needed. Arnica montana gel is also applied to the forehead and temple areas hourly in the first day postoperative and 3–5 times daily in the subsequent 3–4 days. This regimen, along with perioperative steroids and application of ice packs, has resulted in much lower rates of swelling and bruising in the author's practice.

Patients who do not require general anesthesia (the majority of patients) are told to have a good breakfast prior to arriving at the office. They are also asked to avoid caffeine and heavy exercise the night before and the morning of surgery. Peri-operative antibiotics are prescribed.

ANESTHESIA

This author gives a fairly generous dose of preoperative sedation, as dictated by the patient's weight, past drug exposure, and personal preferences. The surgical day is long and patients can be quite anxious. Anxiety, in turn, affects the patient's ability to tolerate even a small amount of discomfort. Thus, oral medications include 10–20 mg diazepam orally (PO), 1–2 mg lorazepam PO, and 5 mg vicodin PO. After the intravenous (IV) line is inserted, 60 mL blood is withdrawn for use in platelet-rich plasma (PRP) and then lactated ringers are given to help hydrate the patient. This IV line can then be used to add

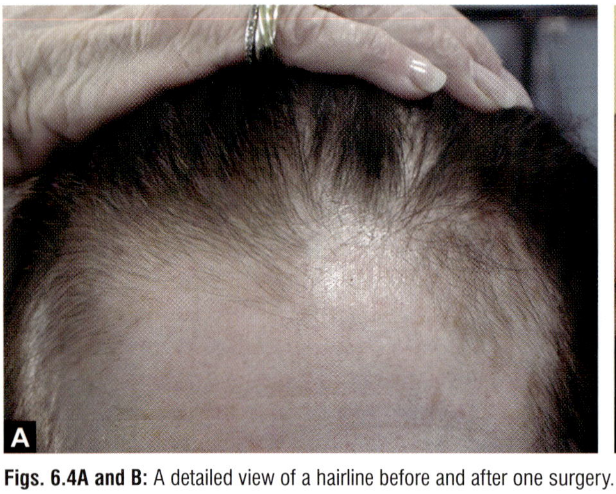

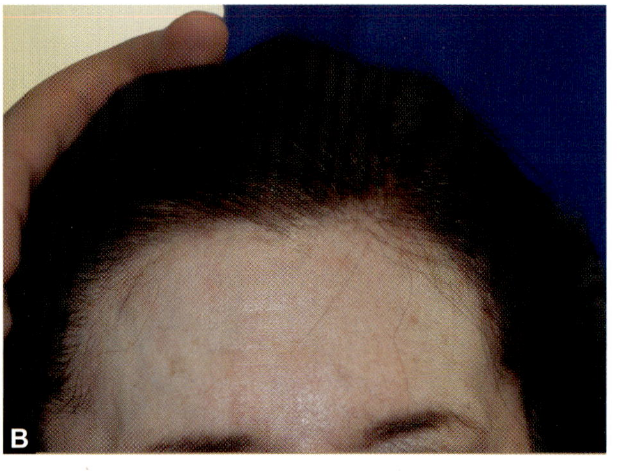

Figs. 6.4A and B: A detailed view of a hairline before and after one surgery.

additional medications as needed. Decadron 8 mg IV is given in two divided doses during the morning to help reduce postoperative swelling.

If the patient has expressed extreme anxiety about the initial injections of local anesthesia then fentanyl 25-50 μg and/or midazolam 1–2 mg can be added through the IV line. Throughout the day sedation can be tailored as needed. In most cases, the morning dose of medications lasts throughout the day. If the patient becomes restless in the afternoon, an IV dose of 50 mg diphenhydramine will often help her fall asleep. Each patient should receive at least one liter of IV fluid throughout the day, and patients with lower blood pressure may need a second liter. The extra fluid does have a truly beneficial effect on patients in the first night postoperatively.

A solution of 20 cc of lidocaine 2% without epinephrine is mixed with 0.2 mg of epinephrine 1/1,000 to create a solution with 1/100,000 epinephrine. The stock solution of lidocaine with epinephrine is more acidic and, therefore, stings more than a freshly prepared solution. There are also more female patients who report an extreme sensitivity to epinephrine and this allows the author to titrate the concentration. The epinephrine solution used for vasoconstriction is a 1/100,000 solution of normal saline and epinephrine. In most female cases, this author utilizes very little of this epinephrine solution (0–8 cc), preferring to use plain normal saline instead. When injected very superficially in the dermis (3 cc syringe and 30G needle), the normal saline provides mechanical compression of the vessels thus minimizing bleeding, and also helps separate the follicles of the pre-existing hair facilitating site creation. Bupivacaine 0.05% without epinephrine is used to reinforce the ring blocks.

Although never proven in a randomized controlled study, the author hypothesizes that generous use of epinephrine in hair transplant procedures may contribute to greater postoperative telogen effluvium. The ring block is performed in stages, and gradually, so that the initial wheals are anesthetized fully before they are used to advance the solution laterally. It is very important to try to avoid the female patients' more superficial vasculature. If a bruise begins developing early on the procedure day, arnica gel is applied to the nearby area intraoperatively.

For patients reporting anesthesia that "wore off early" in past surgical or dental procedures, the initial ring block is performed with 3% or even 4% lidocaine with 1/50,000 epinephrine. Often a much smaller quantity will achieve much faster and long-lasting results in these patients, who frequently have green in their eyes, freckles, or red hair.[7] Occasionally, the author will use a supraorbital block with 2% lidocaine without epinephrine. This method is utilized in patients who have extensive superficial vasculature or have bruised very badly in the past. The author may also choose to use this intraoperatively, if there is excessive bleeding and the anesthesia has become ineffective within a short time of administration.

DONOR HARVEST

For women, the surface area and location of optimal donor hair often vary from men. Some women have a donor area located further inferiorly than might be expected and some have good donor even above the ears. There is also less worry about vertex thinning as occurs in men. The donor should be evaluated for the degree of miniaturization in order to properly advise the patient about the longevity of some of the transplanted hair (Fig. 6.5). Women with extensive miniaturization should be cautioned about diminished results over time. The majority of them still feel that having a fuller head of hair during their younger years outweighs the potential risk of thinning later.

Unified Tissue Extraction

The donor area in female hair restoration is usually removed as a unified tissue extraction or strip.

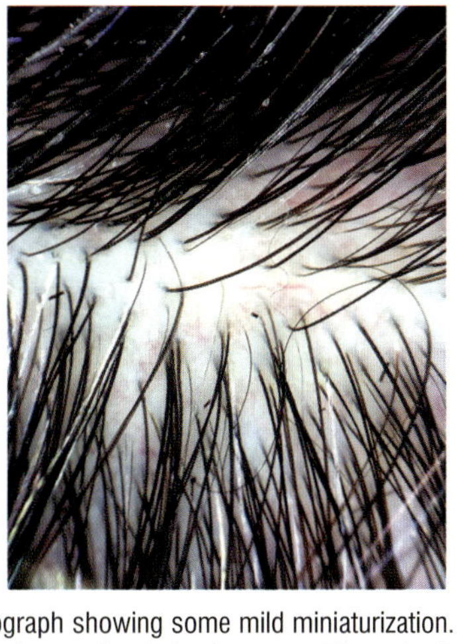

Fig. 6.5: Photograph showing some mild miniaturization. This dermatoscope photograph was taken in the donor area. The patient's age (57 years) makes this less concerning. Nonetheless, the photograph was shown to the patient to help explain to her the impact of higher caliber hair, and that although the transplanted hair is more permanent than most of the existing hair in the area, some of it is not permanent and will be lost over time.

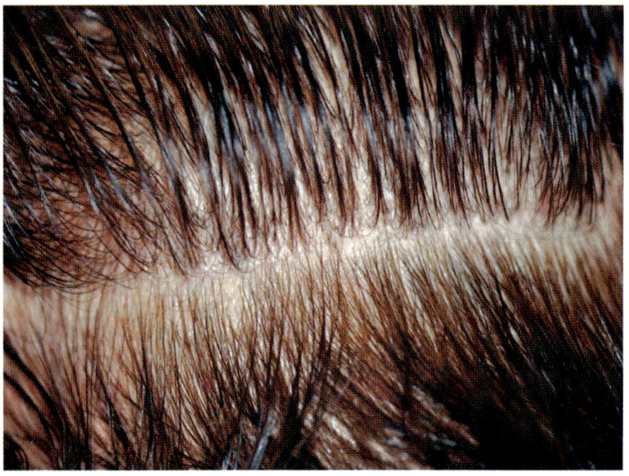

Fig. 6.6: A close-up photograph of a typical donor scar in a woman after unified tissue extraction. The patient reported that her hairstylist cannot "even find where the grafts were taken from"—a not uncommon remark.

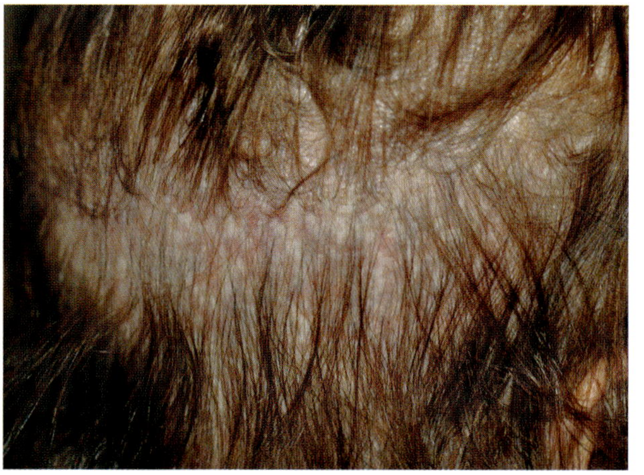

Fig. 6.7: A photograph of the donor area in a woman who had two follicular unit extraction (FUE) procedures performed by another doctor. Note the punctuate scars and generally thinned look of the remaining hair. The patient presented to me looking for more density in the recipient area, as she felt there was limited improvement after the FUE; however, her donor area has been depleted.

The area is sutured in either a single or double layer closure. Most women have fairly thin dermis, so a single layer is sufficient. The 3.0 supramid is used to approximate the wound edges with as little tension as possible. If the donor strip is limited to 10–15-mm width then there is usually no tension. This can also involve taking a wider section centrally and narrowing the strip more laterally. The use of a towel clip to approximate the edges in the tightest region prior to starting the closure can also be helpful. If a double layer closure is deemed necessary the author now uses a 3.0 polydioxanone suture (PDS) (Ethicon PDS II on 26 mm 1/2c reverse cutting needle). The donor scar is usually very difficult to locate even on close inspection (Fig. 6.6).

Follicular Unit Extraction

Follicular unit extraction (FUE) has a major advantage in male patients because they can wear their hair in virtually any style, including a very short "buzz cut". The author has yet to meet a female patient who is concerned with this potential advantage. The other advantage is that the surgeon can cherry-pick the desired size of FUs, which is beneficial treating smaller specialized regions. Follicular unit extraction may also be a good option for women with very tight scalps or who are fearful of the postoperative pain from a strip harvest.

The major disadvantage of FUE for women is that the entire donor area must be shaved. This can take several years to regrow. There are also concerns about graft survival with FUE and women already have significant donor hair limitations. Long hair FUE can be utilized, but this, usually, is considerably more expensive and yields fewer grafts.[9] Perhaps, most importantly, FUE actually leaves the donor area looking less dense, creating a potential problem where none previously existed (Fig. 6.7).

RECIPIENT SITE CREATION AND GRAFT SIZES

The creation of recipient sites is intricately tied to one's decision about graft sizes, as well as an evaluation of both the donor tissue and the recipient area. The author uses a variety of graft sizes, including single FU grafts (one-haired, two-haired, 3+hair, FF), double follicular unit grafts and even triple follicular unit (TFU) grafts. The corresponding tools for recipient site creation include various gauge needles, blades cut to size and even occasionally hollow-core round sites (0.9–1.17 mm in size).

The initial plan regarding graft size is based upon the pattern and distribution of thinning hair in the recipient area, and what variation of graft size is likely to create the greatest illusion of density. The hairline is always done in a very irregular pattern with single FUs and an increasing gradient of 1–3 hairs. The technicians in the office also grade the grafts according to how fine the hairs are within the FU and finer haired grafts are utilized in the most anterior aspect of the hairline. The transitions between the sizes of graft within the transplanted area should also be irregular. Some patients have very discrete areas of atrichia further posterior to the hairline that can be removed with a hollow-core instrument (a slot or round punch) and replaced with a TFU (Figs. 6.8A and B).

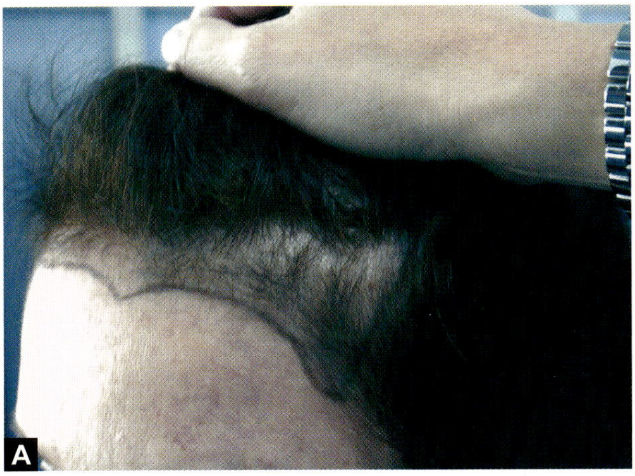

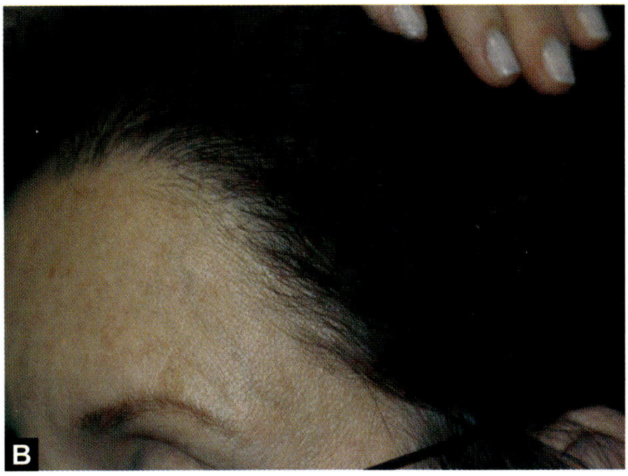

Figs. 6.8A and B: Photographs showing the surgical pattern and results achieved by utilizing multifollicular unit to create areas of higher density while trying to still cover a reasonably sized region.

Upon microscopic evaluation of the entire donor area, it may become evident that the hair within the tissue is not appropriate for the previously chosen size of graft. The donor FUs may be spaced too far apart to make a reasonably sized multifollicular unit graft. There may be very few naturally occurring multihaired FUs. Alternatively, testing of the grafts in the recipient area may make the surgeon change the choice of graft size or site size, because the tissue has almost no elasticity, or there is no recoil of the tissue or a different size site makes the placing of the grafts less traumatic.[10] This interplay of factors underlies the importance of good communication between the physician and her team of assistants.

The required density and distribution of sites will depend on the size of the area requiring treatment, the amount of pre-existing hair, and the spacing between those hairs. For women, high-density grafting can lead to more significant telogen effluvium postoperatively and is not usually recommended. As a general rule, the larger the size site, the lower the density should be—*see* Table 6.2 for details. The photos included in this article have all been accomplished with these densities.

One of the most important factors in the success of female hair transplant surgery is the ability of the surgeon to follow the angle and direction of the existing hair (Figs. 6.9A to C). This results in the most natural appearance and helps to create the illusion of density. There are actually three vectors to be aware of: the right–left orientation, the acuteness of the angle of exit from the scalp and the tilt or lean of the graft. When creating sites at the correct angle, there is a smooth tactile sensation, whereas an erroneous angle will produce slightly more resistance and a gritty sensation. The pre-existing hair needs to be protected both on the surface of the scalp and from transection within the epidermis or dermis. Occasionally, patients who have had surgery elsewhere will report in the consultation that they had virtually immediate loss of hair after the procedure. It is the author's opinion that the surgeon likely *cut* the hair very close to the scalp or transected hairs and this resulted in a thinner look almost instantaneously.

Table 6.2: General guidelines for site size and density.
One haired FU—0.7-mm blade or 20G needle at 25–35 FU/cm²
Two haired FU—0.9-mm blade or 19G needle at 20–30 FU/cm
3+ hair FU—1.0-mm blade at 15–25 FU/cm
DFU or TFU—blade or hollow core sized according to graft at 10–15 FU/cm

It is important to test grafts in the sites, before too many have been created. Additionally, different regions of the scalp may respond differently. The scalps of patients who have had previous surgery or who have a fibrotic feel to the tissue very often have very little *give* to the tissue, meaning that there is resistance when trying to dilate the site. At the same time, the tissue does not spring back after graft insertion—a characteristic the author refers to as *no recoil*. These patients are known in the practice as "difficult plants". The solution is not always clear; a larger site will be easier to open, but the graft will slip out more easily. The use of superficial saline injection in the area can sometimes help reduce slipping. Sometimes the sites need to be spaced further apart. In extreme cases, a stick and place technique may be the best option.

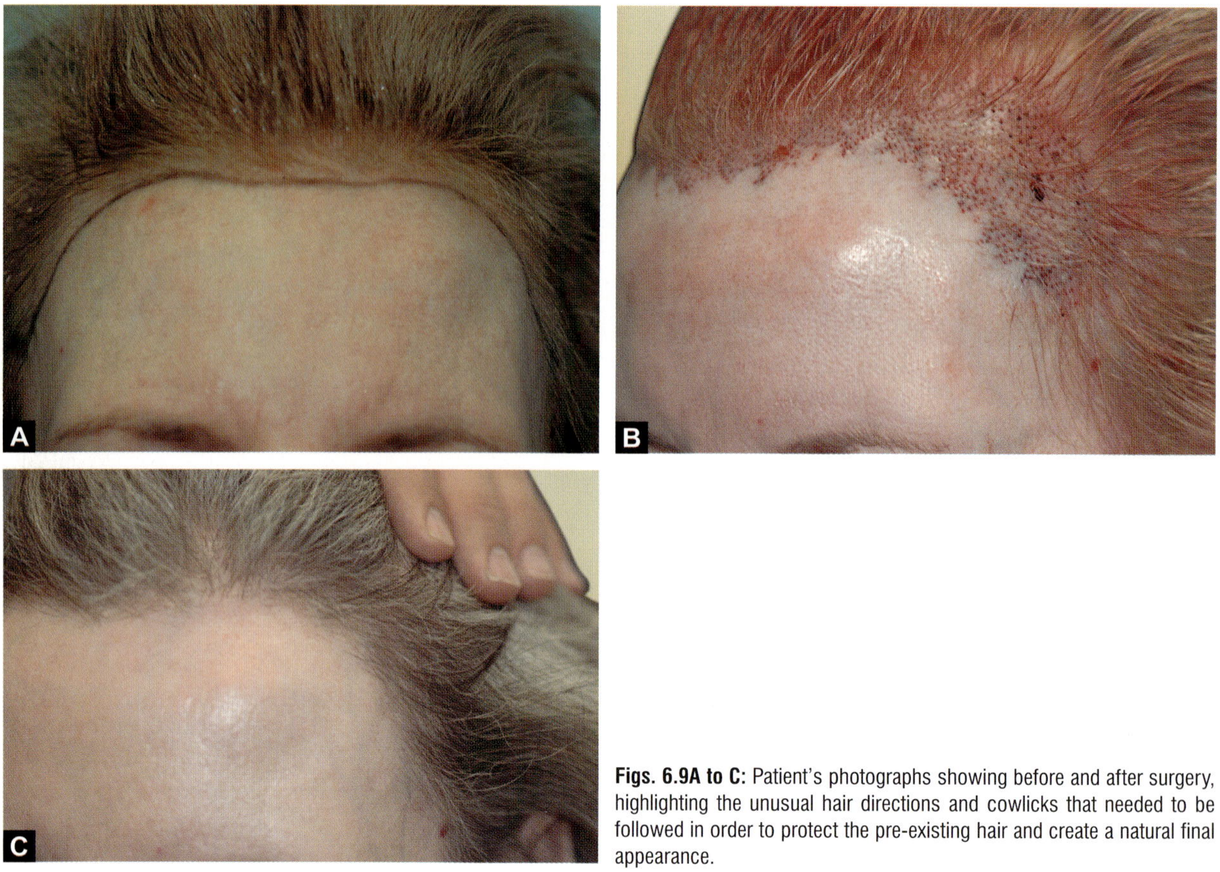

Figs. 6.9A to C: Patient's photographs showing before and after surgery, highlighting the unusual hair directions and cowlicks that needed to be followed in order to protect the pre-existing hair and create a natural final appearance.

SPECIAL CONSIDERATIONS AND TECHNIQUES

Female Patients Postrhytidectomy or Browlift

Many female patients present for hair transplant surgery following plastic surgery in order to improve upon their final result. The main concern usually is a thin linear scar in the hair-bearing region that requires a small session of grafts. Hair transplant surgery into scar tissue requires that the surgeon assess the vascular supply carefully as surgery proceeds. Some areas of the scar may have a good blood supply, allowing for a normal density of sites to be created. More often there is a reduced blood supply and the recipient sites have to be created at much lower densities, requiring the need for a second small surgical procedure. In addition, some scars are fairly hypo-pigmented and this color difference may still be noticeable after hair transplantation. In these patients a flesh colored tattooing can be performed to make the scar more uniform with the patient's skin color.[11]

Other women present after facial plastic surgery with an alteration in their hairline contour superiorly, laterally or in the periauricular region. Hair transplant procedures for these patients are generally more extensive and may simultaneously address regions just posterior to the hairline that have also been affected by FPHL. The surgical treatment of these patients follows similar surgical planning in women presenting with FPHL involving the frontotemporal regions, with the addition of the preauricular (and sometimes supra-auricular or postauricular) areas. In most patients one surgery is sufficient, although a second smaller procedure may be necessary to increase the density in the region of the scar itself. The results are excellent and help complete the process of facial rejuvenation started by the plastic surgeon (Fig. 6.10).

Platelet-rich Plasma

Platelet-rich plasma has become a popularly touted treatment for hair loss in recent years. Unfortunately, there are no large controlled trials to prove its efficacy.[12] One recent pilot study suggested a 40% efficacy but there are still many unknowns about optimal concentration and duration of efficacy after treatment.[13]

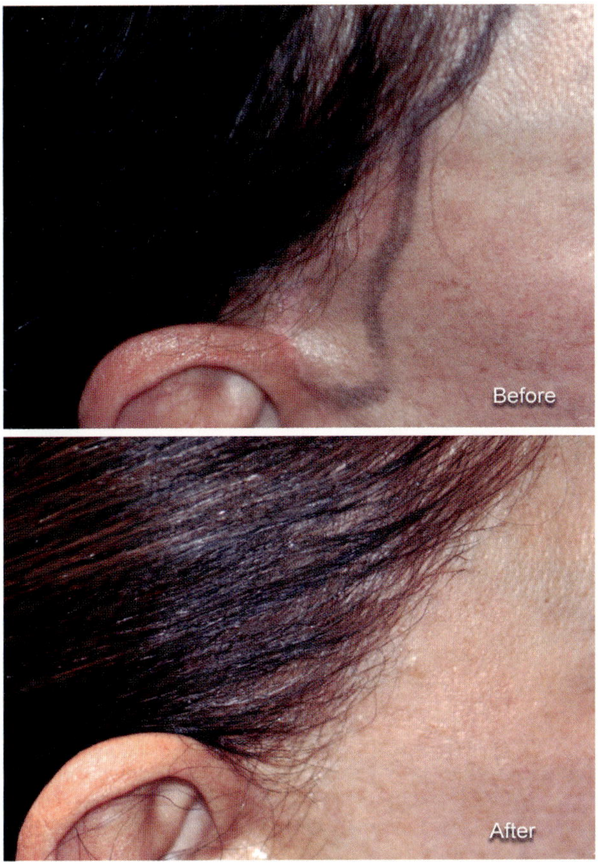

Fig. 6.10: A female patient post-facelift presented for hair transplant surgery to help camouflage some of the surgical scars and recreate her hairline contour. Although the hypopigmentation of the scar is still somewhat visible after the hair transplant, it is much less noticeable. In some patients in whom this is a significant issue a tattoo artist can create camouflage preoperatively with a pigment that matches the skin color (not the hair color).

Several years ago, the author began using PRP as part of every surgical procedure. At the start of the surgical day 60 cc of blood is drawn and processed into PRP, generally producing 5–7 cc for use. The PRP is combined with ACell MatriStem Micromatrix (Acell Inc., Columbia, MD) which is a sterile, porcine-derived extracellular matrix that has been shown to improve wound healing.[14] This solution is used to bathe grafts prior to insertion into the scalp and if there is a sufficient quantity, a portion is injected into an area not being treated with hair transplant surgery.

It was the author's intention to study the potential beneficial effects of this. Unfortunately, it is exceptionally difficult to ascertain a difference in hair counts or hair caliber in patients with pre-existing hair and ongoing loss of that hair. It is necessary to try to design a more reliable study protocol to examine the effects in these patients. Nonetheless, the use of PRP and ACell has continued because the author has observed a slight increase in the speed of recovery and growth of the transplanted hair. A new study could be designed to investigate that potential advantage alone.

Pearls to Practically Manage Hair Transplantation with Long Hair

Women with long hair pose additional technical difficulties for the surgeon and staff. Several techniques have helped to manage this challenge. First, patients are asked to wash their hair in the morning prior to surgery. Betadine is used to further clean the scalp prior to beginning. During the donor removal, it is ideal to use one or two hair ties that can be fashioned out of surgical tape folded in half lengthwise. The hair superior to the donor area is tied above the donor, and depending on how much hair exists, a second tie can be used for the hair inferiorly. Any hairs that get trapped under the suture line need to be extricated, so that the patient does not pull on the suture line when brushing her hair after surgery.

The hair in the recipient area provides a guide regarding the direction and angle at which the sites need to be created. However, it can also get easily tangled and then combing becomes difficult and/or pulls out existing hair. To manage this problem our team uses a wide-toothed comb, sterile water-based gel (close to the scalp) and conditioner for the distal ends of the hair.

POSTOPERATIVE CARE

The author has fairly involved postoperative instructions. Although other surgeons may have success without these precautions, the author believes that good postoperative care is largely responsible for the *consistency* of the patient results.

Immediate Care

Patients have a bandage overnight and are seen the following morning for bandage removal, graft check and a first hair washing by an experienced technician. This helps start the postoperative week with minimal blood and crusting. It also gives the patient the opportunity to ask questions about the postoperative care. Patients are told that if any sign or symptom occurs that is not described in the written postoperative instructions,[15] to *not* assume it is normal. They are

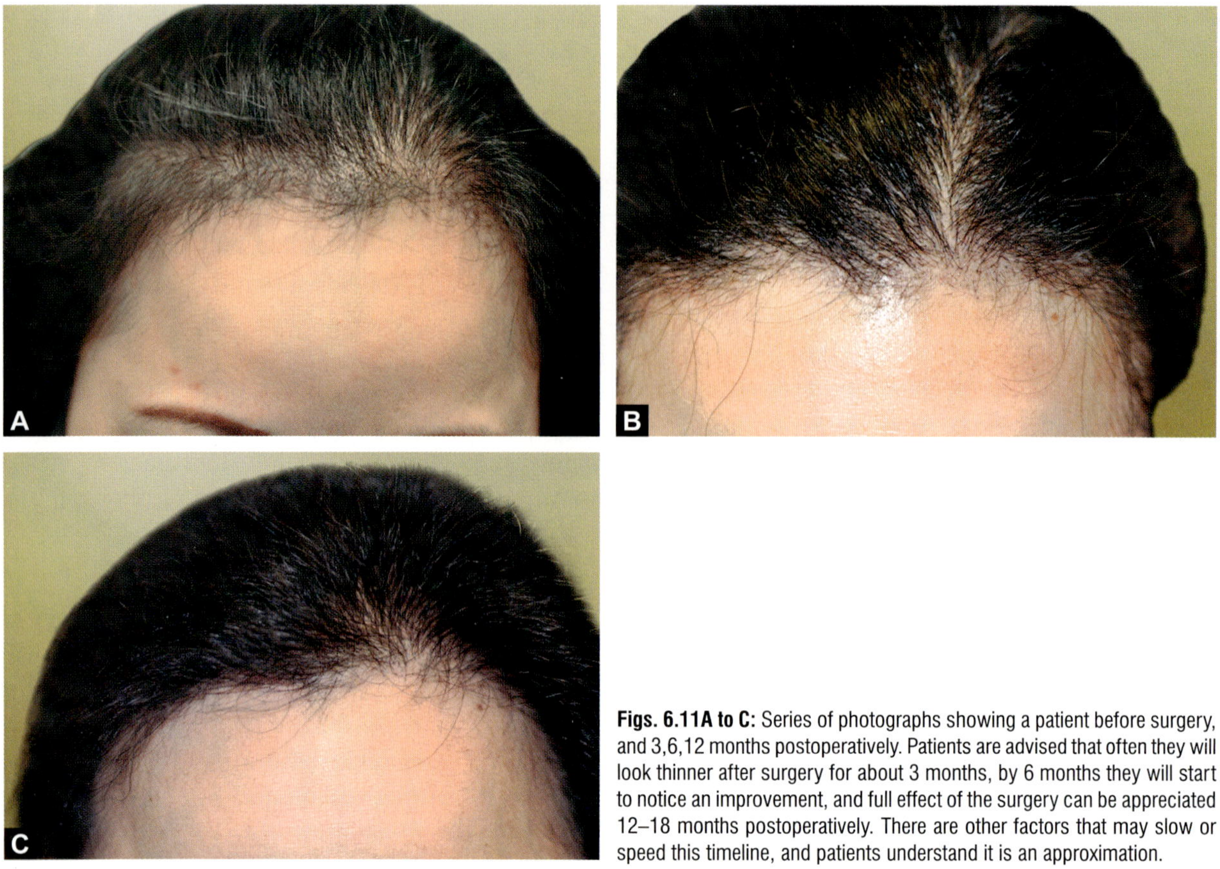

Figs. 6.11A to C: Series of photographs showing a patient before surgery, and 3,6,12 months postoperatively. Patients are advised that often they will look thinner after surgery for about 3 months, by 6 months they will start to notice an improvement, and full effect of the surgery can be appreciated 12–18 months postoperatively. There are other factors that may slow or speed this timeline, and patients understand it is an approximation.

instructed to call the office or to come in to have it checked. There is an open-door policy after surgery and patients can come for as much or as little reassurance as necessary. Most patients come to the office for three postoperative appointments: for bandage removal, a mid-week check and suture removal.

Intermediate Follow-up

All patients return for follow-up 4-6 weeks after surgery. During this visit, the patient is assessed for additional postoperative sequelae including telogen effluvium, folliculitis, and donor area inflammation. Although the occurrence of telogen effluvium only requires reassurance, this is very helpful to the patient. If there is folliculitis, it may or may not need treatment with antibiotics or steroids. Inflammation in the donor area is indicated by local erythema, a raised scar, or itching. It is treated with intralesional kenalog 3.33 mg/mL at the time of the appointment and two to three additional injections at 3-week intervals. This regimen and follow-up have ensured exceptional consistency in the donor scars.

Final results from the hair transplant can be seen 12–18 months after surgery, although occasionally may be appreciated earlier (Figs. 6.11A to C). Patients are encouraged to come for this final postoperative visit to assess the results and take postoperative photos for future reference. It also helps ensure the surgeon remains enthusiastic and energized by the patient's satisfaction and appreciation!

CONCLUSION

Female hair transplantation continues to evolve and produces undetectable natural results that improve the quality of patients' lives. At this point in time, surgery is the only available method to reliably restore hair in women suffering from hair loss. Responsibly devised surgical plans, with consideration of future areas of loss, help ensure long-term results. Ideally, surgery is combined with medical therapy to slow the ongoing loss and potentially reverse some of the miniaturization that has occurred. Hopefully, in the future surgery will be combined with other more successful modalities and medical treatments.

REFERENCES

1. Unger W, Unger R. Hair transplanting: an important but often forgotten treatment for female pattern hair loss. J Am Acad Dermatol. 2003;49:853-60.
2. Unger W. Candidacy of females for hair transplantation. Hair Transplant Forum Int. 2011;21(4): 105-12.
3. Rogers, N. Imposters of androgenetic alopecia: diagnostic pearls for the hair restoration surgeon. In: Konior R, Gabel S (Eds). Hair Restoration. Facial Plas Surg Clin North Am 2013;21(3):325-34.
4. Rudnicka L, Olszewska M, Rakowska A (Eds). Atlas of Trichoscopy. London: Springer; 2012.
5. Tosti A. Dermoscopy of Hair and Scalp Disorders with Clinical and Pathological Correlations. London: Informa Healthcare; 2007.
6. Unger R, Wesley C. Technical and philosophical approaches influencing perceptions of female candidacy and results in hair restoration surgery—Treatment Strategies. Dermatology. 2011;1(1):142-5.
7. Unger W. The pre-operative phase. In: Unger W, Shapiro R, Unger R, Unger M (Eds). Hair Transplantation, 5th edition. New York: Informa Healthcare; 2011. pp. 198-212.
8. Unger R. Female hair restoration. In: Konior R, Gabel S (Eds). Hair Restoration. Facial Plast Surg Clin North Am. 2013;21(3):407-13.
9. Cole J, Insalaco C. State-of-the-art FUE: advanced non-shaven technique. Hair Transplant Forum Intl. 2014;24(5):161-9.
10. Wolf B. The art and craft of recipient site creation and graft placement. Hair Transplant Forum Intl. 2014;24(2):41-9.
11. Unger W, Unger R, Wesley C. The surgical treatment of cicatricial Alopecia. Dermatol Ther. 2008;21(4): 295-311.
12. Jimenez F. Platelet rich plasma (PRP) in patients with androgenetic alopecia (AGA): does it work? Hair Transplant Forum Intl. 2014;24(1):5-6.
13. Schiavone G, Raskovic D, Greco J, et al. Platelet-rich plasma for androgenetic alopecia: a pilot study. Dermatol Surg. 2014;40:1010-9.
14. Mayresh, U. Novel wound healing technologies: a review. Int'l J Pharm Sc Rev Res. 2011;10(2);article-012:.64-6.
15. Parsley W, Waldman M. Management of the post-operative period. In: Unger W, Shapiro R, Unger R, Unger M (Eds). Hair Transplantation, 5th edition. New York: Informa Healthcare; 2011. pp. 416-8.

CHAPTER

7

Corrective Hair Transplantation

Nicole Rogers, Craig Ziering

INTRODUCTION

It is essential for hair surgeons to know how to revise poor cosmetic outcomes from prior hair transplantation. They may need to address large punch grafts, low hairlines, blunted temporal recessions, or large or unsightly donor scars. Because male and female pattern hair loss is both chronic and progressive, patients who undergo surgery at a young age without medical therapy may be unhappy if they require additional surgeries later on. Other patients may not be interested in further surgery, and may request simple removal of the hair in the grafted areas. It can take skill as well as diplomacy to make patients happy and give them optimal results given their starting point.

HISTORY

Unfortunately, dense, blunted hairlines, and "pluggy" results were the norm during most of the latter half of the 20th century. While temporoparietal flaps like the Juri and Elliot flaps provided coverage in the frontal hairline, they did not look natural. Large 4-mm punch "cornrows" left patients with depleted donor areas and Barbie-doll-looking hair in the frontal scalp. Likewise, grafts were often placed too perpendicularly, leaving a picket-fence appearance.

Leaders in the field of hair transplantation soon identified these issues and developed new ways to make the results more favorable. When Dr Bobby Limmer described the use of stereoscopic magnification to create 1-4 hair follicular units in 1994,[1] it illuminated a path for other surgeons like Manfred Lucas, James Vogel, and Robert Bernstein to further refine the techniques of corrective hair surgery.[2-6] Since then the field of hair transplantation has evolved quickly toward natural and undetectable results.

CONSULTATION

First, one must ascertain the patient's goals. The conservative surgeon should not assume that the patient's concerns will match his or her own. It is helpful to have two mirrors available so that the patient can point out problem areas in the front and/or vertex, if necessary. One should carefully document what hair surgery was done in the past and how many grafts/plugs were placed. It is helpful to examine the donor area carefully to see what hair is available for further surgery and if any wide scarring or keloid exists.

One should also differentiate whether the hair positioning or angle bothers the patient or if they dislike textural skin changes around the grafts. If the patient is willing, take careful photographs for surgical planning. It may also be helpful to upload these to a larger screen to explain what options they have for revision. Try to offer solutions that would include surgical as well as nonsurgical options. For instance, they may benefit from fractional laser resurfacing to address surface irregularities (Fig. 7.1A and B) before undergoing more hair surgery or the more permanent step of graft removal or laser hair removal (LHR).

Finally, one should not disparage other surgeons' work, for fear of making the patient more self-conscious or worsening their self-esteem. Control expectations by planning for two or more sessions to achieve the

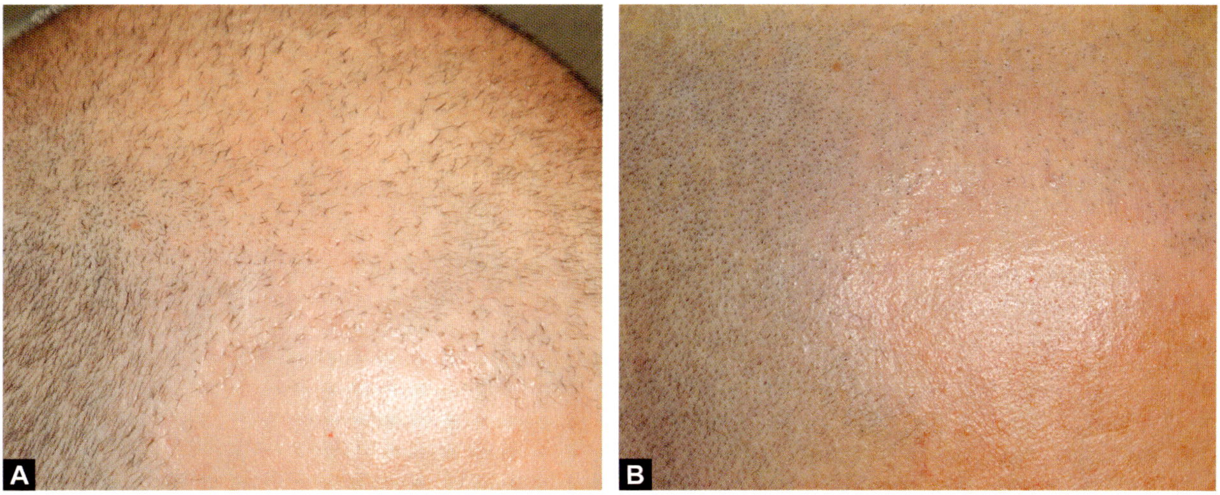

Figs. 7.1A and B: (A) 37-year-old male complaining of textural irregularities after hair transplant surgery with Neograft. (B) Same patient after undergoing fractional laser treatment, now pleased with results.
Courtesy: Mary Lupo MD.

patient's goals. If significant graft recycling is necessary, one may need to transplant closely into the sutured areas where grafts were removed. The grafts may not take well until the initial healing has taken place.

CORRECTION OF RECIPIENT AREA GRAFTING

Plug Grafts in Anterior Scalp

Plug grafts were the most common technique used for hair transplantation in the United States from the 1950s until the late 1980s. It was popularized by dermatologist Norman Orentreich,[7] and while it provided good density in the short run, the grafted areas became highly noticeable after surrounding areas thinned. This was especially problematic prior to the introduction of oral finasteride, which can help slow hair loss and even regrow hairs around the grafted area.

Patients have several options for repair of these oversized punch grafts. Swinehart observed that it is difficult to camouflage these plugs by simply placing smaller grafts in front of them.[8] Lucas described using a 1.5–1.7-mm punch biopsy instrument to partially excise the plugs and allow the small circular wounds to heal secondarily.[2] Vogel slightly modified the technique to use a 3.5-mm punch to remove most of the traditionally sized 4-mm punch grafts, and generally would suture the wounds closed to reduce serous seepage.[4] He coined the term "plug reduction and recycling," and published his results after revising over 100 patients.

Since then it has become quite popular to use local anesthesia and punch trephines to remove the oversized grafts, apply magnification to separate them into individual follicular units, and then replace them back into areas of hair thinning (Figs. 7.2A and B). Good closure of the defects can be achieved with a synthetic 4–0 nonabsorbable nylon suture. Various techniques exist for how to do this, such as removing the entire graft, removing just a portion of the graft (to leave behind some hairs), or removing only the center portion of the grafts.[5] This decision can often be made with the patient depending on how much the size of the grafts bothers them.

As the use of these "cornrow" punch grafts has fallen out of favor, there are fewer patients requiring our expertise in these repairs. However, it is essential to maintain the skill set necessary to help make such repairs in order to become masters in the art of hair transplantation.

Low Hairline

Male patients who undergo hair transplant surgery at an early age (20s) may be saddled with a hairline that looks unnaturally low as they enter their 50s and 60s. This can occur if the hairline is placed less than the recommended 8–9 cm above the glabella, or if their hair loss progresses without the benefit of medical therapy. When consulting with virgin hair transplant candidates, it is imperative to remind them that the hairline can always be lowered, but it is quite difficult to raise. The authors encourage patients toward hairlines that will look good in the short run *and the long run,* which occasionally means transplanting

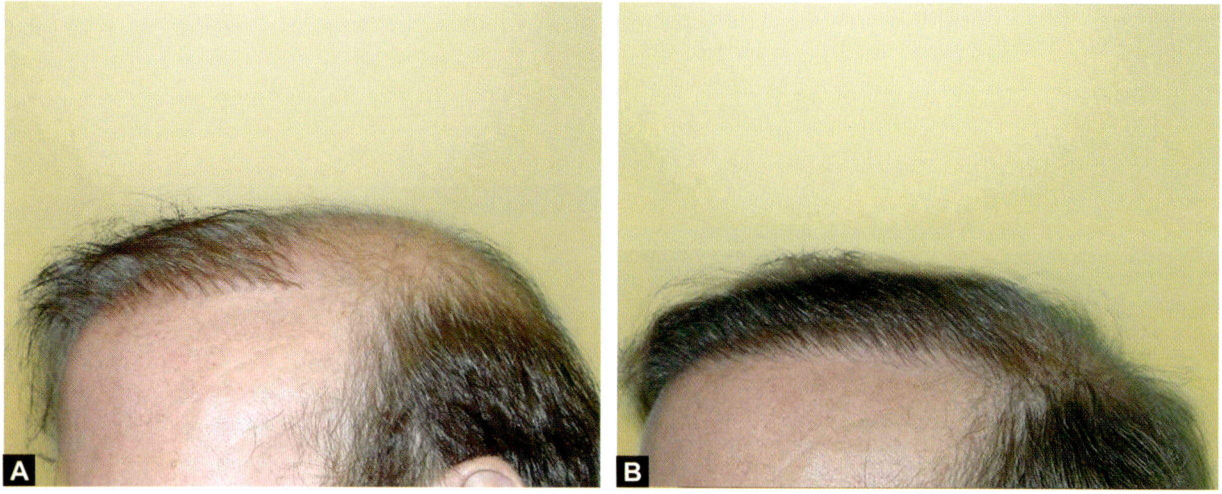

Figs. 7.2A and B: (A) 45 year-old male with oversized punch grafts before. (B) Same patient following graft removal and recycling.

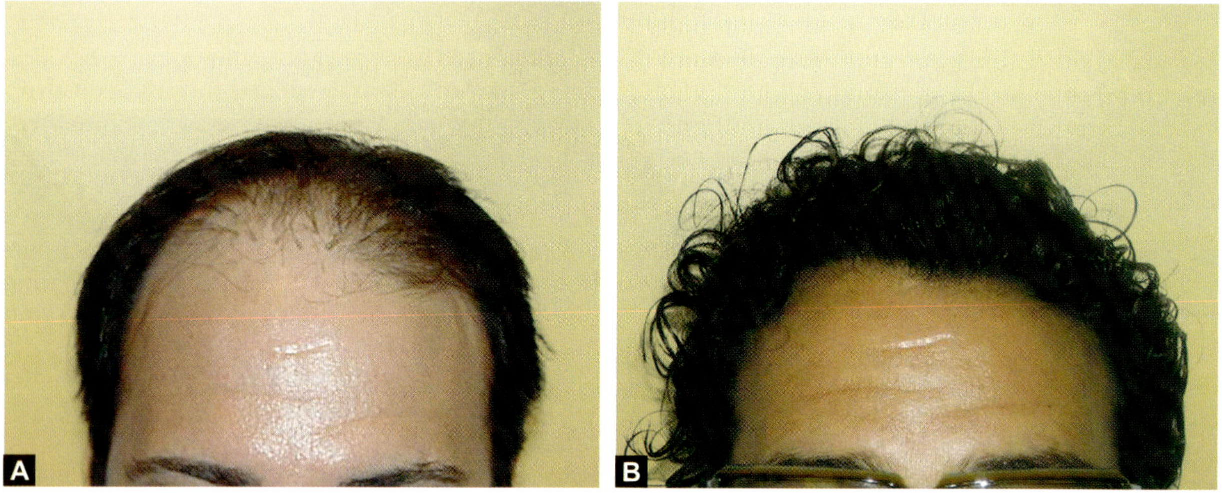

Figs. 7.3A and B: (A) 38-year-old male with oversized punch grafts before. (B) Same patient following graft removal and recycling.

with initial emphasis on the midscalp (Figs. 7.3A and B). That being said, patients with too low a hairline have several options.

The first is to use punch grafts to remove and recycle the grafts as described earlier. The other option is to perform LHR. This is a good option if the patient does not want to undergo further hair surgery and does not want to risk any scarring in the frontal hair line.[9] The patient should understand it can require 6–10 sessions to fully ablate the hair. The best candidates are patients with light skin and dark hair. African-American patients may risk blistering or pigmentary changes because most lasers are less well adapted for hair removal in darker skin types.

Stough described excellent cosmesis using a single linear elliptical harvest of punch grafts.[10] This can offer more reliable hair removal especially in cases where a large number of hairs have been placed too low. One concern is the development of trap-door defect in the more proximal aspect of the scalp. In experienced hands, this technique can be quite helpful.

The issue of a low hairline can be especially troublesome when the temporal recessions are too blunted or rounded. This can leave male patients with a feminine appearance. Ideally these areas should have a masculine, squared-off appearance. If the grafts are oversized, they may be removed and recycled. If the grafts are 1–4 hair single follicular units, it may be difficult to punch them all out without leaving scarring. Laser hair removal may be a better option in such situations.

Incorrect Angling of Grafts

Generally, grafts look most natural when they are placed at a very acute angle toward the midline front of the scalp. Ideally, recipient sites should be placed so that the exiting hairs are at a 30° (or less) angle from the scalp. When larger (3–5-mm) punch grafts were used along the frontal hairline, there often resulted an unnatural angling of the hairs, such that they grew out perpendicular to the scalp surface. This can occur even with smaller mini or micrografts, but may not appear as obvious. Grafts can also appear unnatural if they are placed too radially, angling laterally, and away from the midline.

The correction of these grafts may depend on whether there are just a few isolated grafts or whether there are many (which may require linear excision). Patients may also benefit from LHR if they do not wish to reuse the grafts or risk having any scarring in the area. African-American patients whose skin is too dark for LHR may consider removal with 0.8-mm punch grafts so long as they do not have a history of keloid formation.

Skin Textural Changes

Another unfortunate result of oversized punch grafts can be changes in surrounding skin texture. Reports exist of pitting (if grafts are placed too deeply) or tenting (if grafts are not placed deeply enough). Historically, dermabrasion improves skin texture but can involve pinpoint bleeding and requires careful wound care. More recently, nonablative lasers offer similar corrective capabilities but with less down time.

Avram described the use of a 1450-nm diode laser to treat surface irregularities in a hair transplant patient. This patient presented for cobblestoning around large punch grafts from 1989 and 1992. Despite shaving his head daily, he was still bothered by the uneven skin changes. He underwent 3-month treatment sessions (6-mm spot size, 11.5 J/cm^2 with cryogen for 33 ms). After an additional 3 months, there was clear evidence of improvement in skin texture to both patient and physician (Figs. 7.4A and B).[11] Fractional nonablative laser may also prove useful for addressing skin texture changes due to hair transplantation.

Correction of Indian Filing

Another result of early hair transplantation was the use of slits to create recipient sites. When grafts were placed in these linear slits, they would occasionally get compressed into linear "Indian files". This could be especially noticeable if there was also evidence of concavity or pitting. When dilators were used to stretch the skin, grafts could sink too low after healing and look unnatural as well.

Correction of Vertex Scalp

The decision to transplant the vertex should be approached with caution, because it is difficult to foresee what degree of thinning men will experience there. While it is normal for a man to have thinning in the vertex, it is not normal for men to have an unnatural looking island of transplanted hair there. Most surgeons nowadays are very cautious in their recommendation to treat the crown in patients who

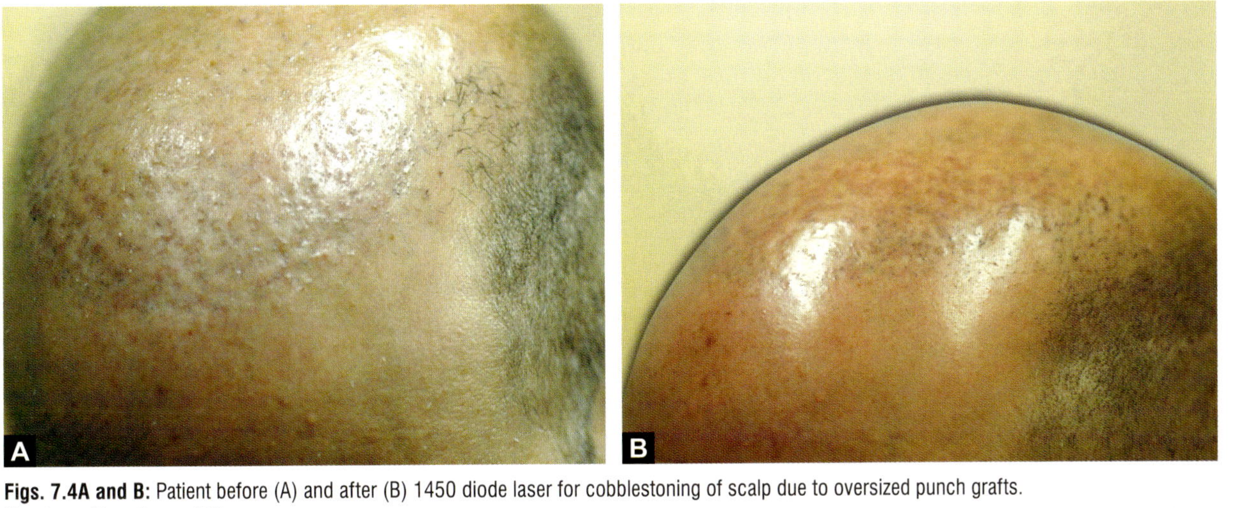

Figs. 7.4A and B: Patient before (A) and after (B) 1450 diode laser for cobblestoning of scalp due to oversized punch grafts.
Courtesy: Marc Avram MD.

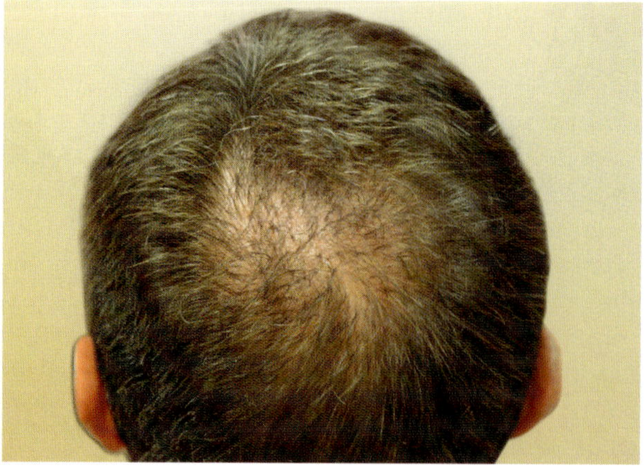

Fig. 7.5: Oversized punch grafts in the vertex.

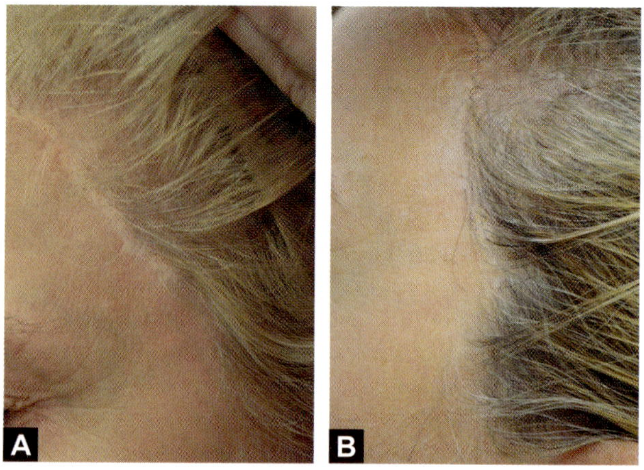

Figs. 7.6A and B: 52 y/o female before (A) and after (B) correction of brow lift scar.

are under 40. Even so, only the anterior crown is transplanted unless the patient is advancing in age and has a well-established pattern of thinning.

For patients who have large pluggy grafts in the vertex, it may be necessary to remove them entirely, either with punch biopsy instrument of the appropriate size or with LHR (Fig. 7.5). This decision will be largely based on whether the patient desires to relocate the grafts to a more anterior part of the scalp or to do away with them altogether.

Facelift and Browlift Scars

As people live longer, facelifts, browlifts, and necklifts have become commonly performed procedures. Modern techniques usually can hide any resulting scars behind the sideburns or ears. There is evidence that minoxidil can also be used prophylactically to reduce this hair loss.[12] However, scars do occasionally result in the sideburn area, along the hairline or behind the ears. To address these, 1–4 hair follicular unit grafts can be successfully placed in these areas (Figs. 7.6A and B).[13] It is essential to use single follicular units, angled acutely in the direction of nearby hairs. Some surgeons are skilled at anticipating such localized hair loss and can perform simultaneous hair transplantation and facial rejuvenation.[14]

Softening of Thick Terminal Hairs

Occasionally, patients present because they do not like the appearance of thick terminal hairs in the area of transplantation. This can occur even with appropriate placement and angling of single follicular unit grafts. It can be especially troublesome in the eyebrow area or along the temporal recessions, which should appear soft. Topical eflornithine cream is approved for the treatment of unwanted facial hair in women. It can be used to soften such existing terminal hairs. The only downside is that it must be used continuously. Others have suggested using LHR to soften a harsh hairline. By limiting the total number of treatments, hairs will miniaturize but not be lost entirely. One surgeon uses follicular unit extraction (FUE) from the nape of the neck to avoid this problem and to obtain soft fine hairs.[15]

CORRECTION OF DONOR AREA

Localized Scarring from Punch Grafts

Prior use of punch grafts can leave the donor area with a scattering of 3–4-mm scars, depending on the size and number of punches harvested. These scars can be especially noticeable when patients are swimming or the hair is wet. For patients desiring further hair transplantation, one can perform a linear ellipse to remove the scar tissue along with new donor hairs in between the donor scars. These hair follicles can then be carefully separated from the scar tissue, under magnification, and then transplanted as 1–4 hair follicular units.

If patients do not need or want additional grafting in the front or vertex, they may undergo FUE to help fill in the neighboring donor scars only. The surrounding areas would be anesthetized locally, and single follicular units would then be harvested using 0.8–1-mm manual or motorized punch biopsy instruments. The donor scars would then be anesthetized and recipient sites would be formed using 18–21 gauge needles. As the surrounding hairs are harvested they can be placed back into the donor "punch" scars.

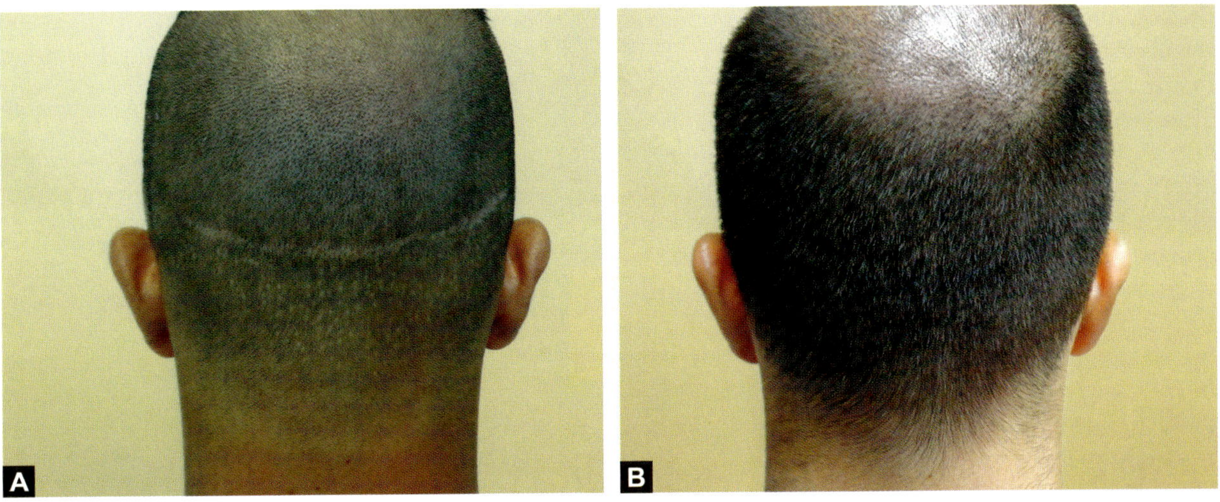

Figs. 7.7A and B: Patient with wide donor scar before (A) and after (B) correction.

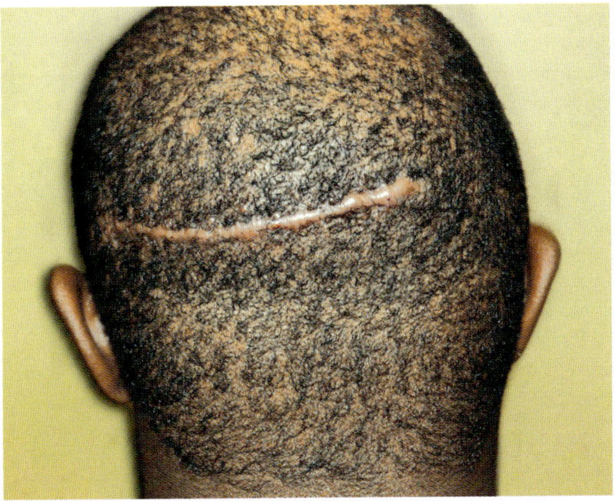

Fig. 7.8: Hypertrophic scar resulting from donor ellipse harvest in a man of African descent.

Wide Donor Scars

Wide donor scars usually result from taking an excessively wide donor ellipse. Occasionally, these scars can be re-excised and successfully heal with a narrower scar (Figs. 7.7A and B). Some colleagues have anecdotally reported increased donor scalp laxity with the injection of hyaluronidase into surrounding donor area (Robert True MD, personal communication Nov. 2014). Others report successfully increasing laxity by instructing patients to stretch the scalp prior to surgery. For patients who do not undergo complete re-excision of the entire donor scar, FUE may also be of benefit. Scalp micropigmentation may also offer camouflaging of the donor scar, but the tattoo pigments used should be carefully based on the age of the patient and any anticipated future thinning (*Do you have any photos of this?*).

In general, the best way to avoid wide donor scars is to keep a conservative width of 1–1.5 cm, especially over the mastoid process. Most patients are willing to undergo repeat surgery when they understand the benefit of gradually allowing the scalp to stretch. They also appreciate having (or attempting to have) the same donor scar used for subsequent procedures.

Keloid Formation

Both keloids and hypertrophic scarring are more common in patients of Caribbean or African ancestry. They are very difficult to treat when they occur in the donor area. The most important goal is to avoid them at all cost, by asking about a keloid history during the consultation. The authors have never seen keloid formation occur in the recipient areas; it is usually in the donor area, and can be worse if the patient undergoes FUE than can result with strip excision (Fig. 7.8). The first-line treatment is generally to inject the keloid with intralesional triamcinolone therapy. Adjunctive therapy can include the application of topical silicone dioxide gel or sheets.[16] Nonablative fractional resurfacing and/or cautious re-excision may also provide some benefit. In patients whose keloid history is ambiguous, it may be wise to start with a small test transplant first.

CONCLUSION

Hair transplantation has evolved considerably over the last 25 years. With appropriate candidate selection, graft angling, and hairline design, modern techniques offer consistently natural-appearing results. Fewer and fewer pluggy results occur now that punch grafts and flaps have fallen out of favor. The use of donor ellipse remains the gold standard, as it allows the production of the greatest number of grafts, from the most permanent donor zone, with the least amount of trauma to the grafts. Follicular unit extraction is an additional way to harvest hair in virgin scalps, and offers a new way to correct donor scars. One caveat is that overzealous use of FUE may eventually require correction as well, if hairs are taken from nonpermanent donor areas. One can only hope that careful study of the past will help avoid further cosmetic mishaps in hair transplantation.

REFERENCES

1. Limmer BL. Elliptical donor stereoscopically assisted micrografting as an approach to further refinement in hair transplantation. J Dermatol Surg Oncol. 1994; 20:789-93.
2. Lucas MW. Partial retransplantation. A new approach in hair transplantation. J Dermatol Surg Oncol. 1994;20:511-4.
3. Lucas MW. Recent advances in hair transplantation. Skin Pharmacol. 1994;7:105-8.
4. Vogel JE. Correction of the cornrow hair transplant and other common problems in surgical hair restoration. Plast Reconstr Surg. 2000;105:1528-36.
5. Bernstein RM, Rassman WR, Rashid N, et al. The art of repair in surgical hair restoration—part I: basic repair strategies. Dermatol Surg. 2002;28:783-94.
6. Bernstein RM, Rassman WR, Rashid N, et al. The art of repair in surgical hair restoration—part II: the tactics of repair. Dermatol Surg. 2002;28:873-93.
7. Orentreich N. Hair transplantation: the punch graft technique. Surg Clin North Am. 1971;51:511-8.
8. Swinehart JM. Hair repair surgery: corrective measures for improvement of older large-graft procedures and scalp scars. Dermatol Surg. 1999;25:523-9.
9. Moreno-Arias GA, Navarra E, Vilalta A, et al. Corrective photoepilation for improper hairline placement after hair transplantation. Dermatol Surg. 2000;26: 790-2.
10. Stough DB. Commentary: Swinehart JM. Hair repair surgery: corrective measures for improvement of older large-graft procedures and scalp scars. Dermatol Surg. 1999;25:523-9.
11. Avram MR, Rogers NE. Use of nonablative laser for corrective hair transplantation. Dermatol Surg. 2009;35:717-8.
12. Eremia S, Umar SH, Li CY. Prevention of temporal alopecia following rhytidectomy: the prophylactic use of minoxidil. A study of 60 patients. Dermatol Surg. 2002;28:66-74.
13. Radwanski HN, Nunes D, Nazima F, et al. Follicular transplantation for the correction of various stigmas after rhytidoplasty. Aesthetic Plast Surg. 2007;31: 62-8.
14. Barrera A. Face lift and hair transplantation as a single procedure. Plast Reconstr Surg. 1999;104:1831-8.
15. Umar S. Eyebrow transplants: the use of nape and periauricular hair in six patients. Dermatol Surg. 2014;40:12.
16. Meaume S, Le Pillouer-Prost A, Richert B, et al. Management of scars; updated practical guidelines and use of silicones. Eur J Dermatol. 2014;24:435-43.

CHAPTER

8

Hair Transplant for the Treatment of Scarring Alopecias

Meena K Singh

INTRODUCTION

The majority of patients who seek consultation for hair restoration are seeking treatment of androgenetic alopecia; however, there is a subset of patients with scarring alopecia who require special consideration for hair restoration. In contrast to the perceived notion that thinning hair is a normal variant of aging, scarring alopecia may often be more cosmetically disfiguring. These patients need special consideration because they not only may be more troubled with the cosmetic appearance of the involved bald areas, but they will also need special technical consideration when performing the surgery.

BACKGROUND

In cicatricial or scarring alopecia, the follicular epithelium has been replaced with fibrous connective tissue. A broader definition, commonly used by hair surgeons, is any form of inflammation or trauma that leads to a scarring process, including hair loss from cosmetic surgery, burns, or radiation.

Cicatricial alopecia is often subdivided into primary and secondary forms. Primary cicatricial alopecia occurs when the hair follicle is the target of the inflammation and disease activity. When the hair follicle just happens to be present in the area of disease activity, such as with radiation dermatitis or burns, this is considered secondary cicatricial alopecia. In this chapter, the approach to hair transplantation of the most common types of cicatricial alopecia will be discussed.

INITIAL EVALUATION

Hair transplantation with scarring alopecia can be more challenging and thus special considerations should be made. Primarily, the inflammatory stage must be inactive in any patient with scarring alopecia considering hair transplantation. Therefore, individuals with scarring alopecia secondary to inflammatory scalp dermatoses should be evaluated and treated medically before surgery can be considered. Most patients will respond within months, but some may take years to become inactive. In addition, the risk of reactivation of the inflammatory stage post-transplant may lead to the loss of the transplanted hairs. It is important to educate patients on the possibility of reactivation so that they understand to seek medical therapy in order to reduce the future graft loss.

Moreover, the patient needs a suitable donor area. Patients with central centrifugal cicatricial alopecia (CCCA), e.g. may have diffuse involvement including the donor region (Fig. 8.1). In addition, scalp fibrosis and diminished blood supply may lead to decreased graft survival, as well as a limited cosmetic outcome.

For these reasons, when a patient with scarring alopecia seeks consultation for hair restoration, accurate diagnosis should be obtained. Consultation may be sought for perceived androgenetic alopecia; however, the patient may truly have a scarring alopecia that clinically mimics androgenetic alopecia (Figs. 8.2A and B). Because transplanting into scarring alopecia takes special considerations, it is pertinent

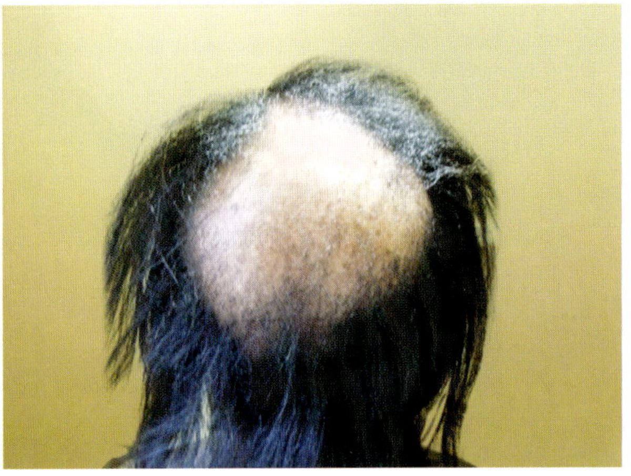

Fig. 8.1: Photograph demonstrating scarring hair loss from central centrifugal cicatricial alopecia involving the donor area.

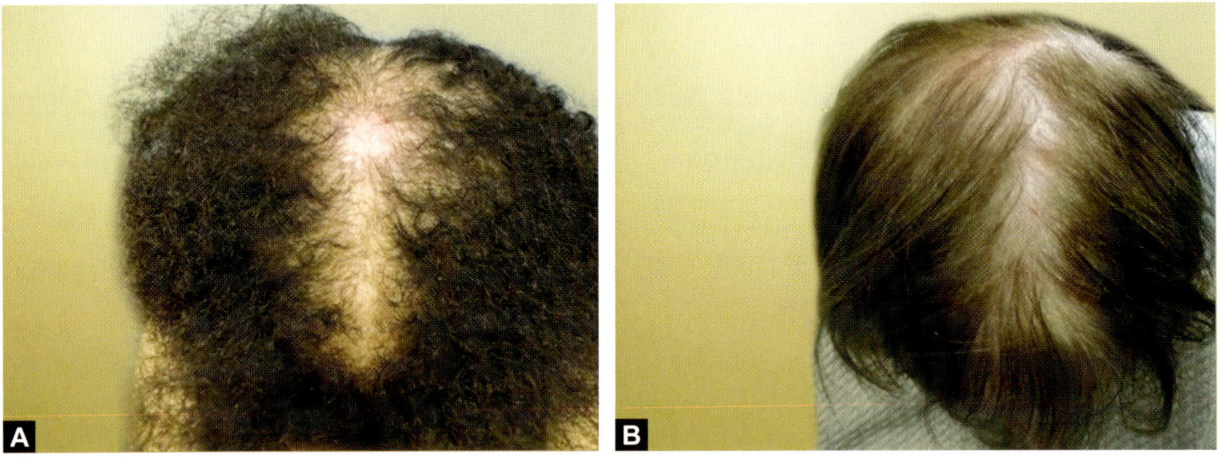

Figs. 8.2A and B: (A) Biopsy-proven central centrifugal cicatricial alopecia mimicking female pattern hair loss. (B) Biopsy-proven lichen planopilaris mimicking female pattern hair loss.

that the surgeon does not miss these diagnoses. The outcomes may be suboptimal, resulting in undesirable cosmetic results and patient dissatisfaction.

Proper diagnosis of cicatricial alopecia entails performing a detailed history and scalp examination (Tables 8.1 and 8.2). Scalp biopsy is strongly recommended. A hair pull test may also be performed to evaluate telogen effluvium. If oozing, bleeding, and/or crusting are present, tissue culture may be warranted.

Table 8.1: Examples of questions to elicit detailed history when diagnosing cicatricial alopecia.

Is the hair loss gradual or sudden?
Is the hair loss shedding or nonshedding?
Is there the presence of high fever or systemic disease?
Is there a recent stressor or medication exposure?
Are there harsh chemicals on hair such as relaxers or dyes?
Is there the presence of itching, burning, tenderness, or oozing?
Is there the history of traumatic hairstyling practices such as tight braids, weaves, or curlers?

HISTOPATHOLOGIC EXAMINATION

When evaluating for cicatricial alopecia, a biopsy can be useful not only to determine the diagnosis but also to determine if the alopecia is end stage and with scarring and perifollicular fibrosis. It is also important to consider where to biopsy, how many biopsies to perform, and how the tissue is processed. The best diagnostic yield is produced when obtaining two biopsies for vertical and horizontal. If direct immunofluorescence is warranted, the vertical section can be bisected using a 15 blade. One piece will be placed in formalin for hematoxylin-eosin staining and the second piece will be placed in media for immunofluorescence, and sent for direct immunofluorescence. Direct immunofluorescence (DIF) is typically performed when either lichen planopilaris (LPP) or lupus erythematosus (LE) is suspected.

PRIMARY CICATRICIAL (SCARRING) ALOPECIA

Primary cicatricial alopecias are inflammatory scalp disorders of largely unknown etiology that lead to areas of permanent, scarring hair loss. The active, inflammatory phases can present with perifollicular erythematous scaly papules, pustules, and bogginess. If left untreated, the chronic inflammation leads to perifollicular fibrosis and the permanent hair loss, likely due to the destruction of the stem cells and sebaceous glands, from ongoing damage to the isthmus of the hair follicle. Once end stage, these inflammatory alopecias can lead to shiny hairless patches with loss of the follicular ostia sometimes with multiple hair follicles exiting one follicular opening, known as "doll hairs".

CLASSIFICATION OF THE PRIMARY CICATRICIAL ALOPECIAS

Based on a proposal from the North American Hair Research Society, primary cicatricial alopecias are further subdivided into three groups on the basis of the type of perifollicular inflammation present: (1) lymphocytic, (2) neutrophilic, and (3) mixed (Table 8.3).

Table 8.2: Examples of scalp examination questions.

Is the hair loss localized or diffuse?
Is there erythema, perifollicular papules, scales, or oozing?
Is there follicular plugging?
Is there cutaneous involvement?
Is there a loss of follicular ostia?
Are there doll hairs present?

The more common types will be discussed below in brief with a focus on the technical considerations needed to transplant.

LYMPHOCYTIC PERIFOLLICULAR INFLAMMATION

Lichen Planopilaris

Lichen planopilaris is a common cause of cicatricial alopecia. In addition, it is a common mimicker of androgenetic alopecia as activity may be subclinical. Lichen planopilaris is more commonly seen in females and Caucasians with scattered patches of partial hair loss, and erythematous, perifollicular scaly papules. This entity is commonly associated with pruritus, burning, and tenderness.

Frontal fibrosing alopecia is thought to be a variant of LPP, typically occurring in postmenopausal women with a band of alopecia in the frontotemporal scalp. A common diagnostic clue is variable perifollicular papules and eyebrow loss.

Lichen planopilaris and frontal fibrosing alopecia (Figs. 8.3A and B) share histopathologic findings with lichenoid interface dermatitis, dyskeratotic keratinocytes at the dermoepidermal junction, and the upper portions of the follicles. Perifollicular fibrosis, scar, and polytrichia may occur at late stages. Examination with direct immunofluorescence demonstrates shaggy fibrin deposition and grouped globular immunoglobulin M (IgM) highlighted adjacent to the follicular epithelium.

CENTRAL CENTRIFUGAL CICATRICIAL ALOPECIA (FURTHER DISCUSSED IN HT IN BLACKS CHAPTER 9)

Central centrifugal cicatricial alopecia is a progressive, expanding, symmetric, scarring hair loss on the crown of the scalp, most commonly seen in

Table 8.3: Proposed classification for primary cicatricial alopecias.

Lymphocytic	*Neutrophilic*	*Mixed*
Chronic cutaneous lupus Erythematosus	Folliculitis decalvans	Acne keloidalis
Lichen planopilaris	Dissecting cellulitis	Acne necrotica
Frontal fibrosing alopecia		Erosive pustular dermatosis
Pseudopalade of Brocq		
Central centrifugal cicatricial alopecia		
Alopecia mucinosa		

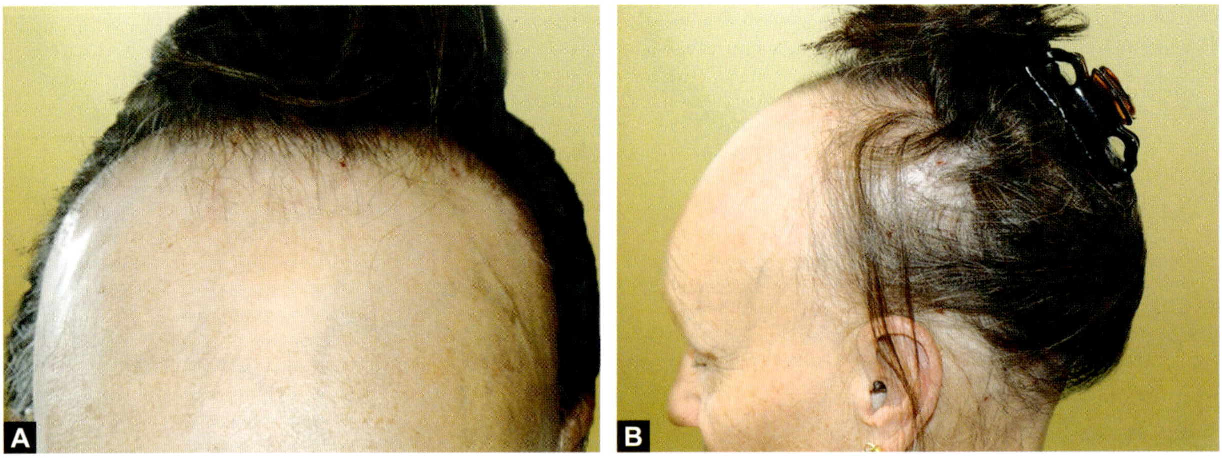

Figs. 8.3A and B: A woman with features of both frontal fibrosing alopecia (A) and lichen planopilaris (B). She demonstrates a wide band like, frontotemporal hairline recession with perifollicular erythematous papules and scarring patches of hair loss throughout the frontal and vertex scalp, as well as eyebrow loss.

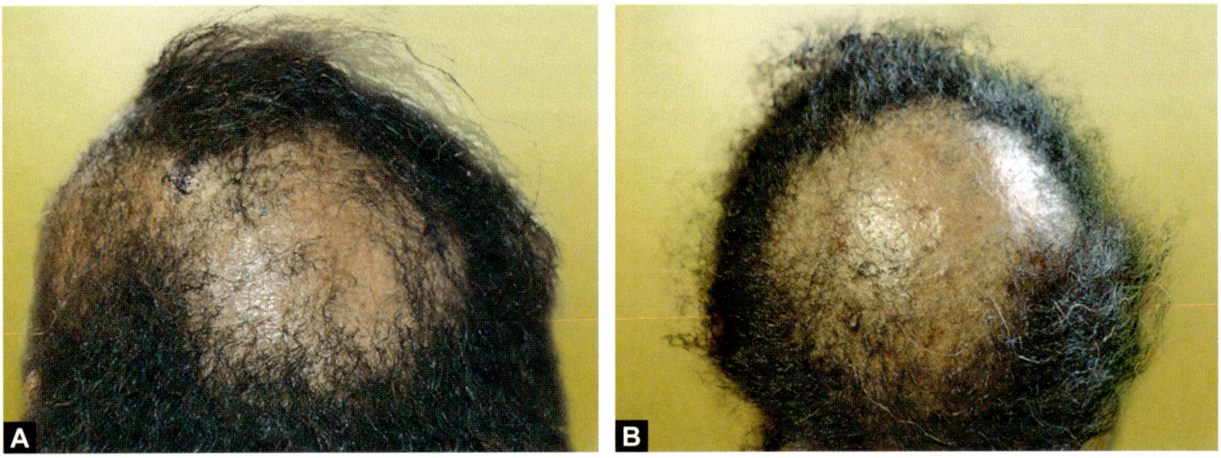

Figs. 8.4A and B: Over the frontoparietal (A) and vertex (B) scalp.

African-American women (Figs. 8.4A and B). Because of the symmetric, progressive nature of this entity, it can often be mistaken for androgenetic alopecia during a hair transplant consultation. On scalp examination, the involved area may appear shiny and atrophic, and doll hairs may be present. Central centrifugal cicatricial alopecia has been variably associated with the use of chemical relaxers and traumatic hairstyling practices such as tight braids, extensions, the use of "hot combs", and permanent relaxers. Histologic examination can demonstrate premature desquamation of the inner root sheath, perifollicular lymphohistiocytic inflammation with variable loss of the sebaceous glands and concentric lamellar fibroplasia. Perifollicular fibrosis and polytrichia may be present in late stages.

Discoid Lupus Erythematosus

When active on the scalp, discoid LE can often present with erythematous to violaceous, hyper/hypopigmented, scaly discoid plaques with follicular plugging (Fig. 8.5). In its end stages, the discoid plaques lead to scarring alopecia with loss of follicular ostia. A clue to diagnosis is hyperpigmented, discoid plaques in the external ear canal. Histopathologic examination reveals hyperkeratosis, follicular plugging, basement membrane thickening, vacuolar interface change, pigment incontinence, dermal mucin deposition, and superficial, deep perifollicular, and perivascular lymphocytic inflammation. Direct immunofluorescence can demonstrate continuous granular deposition with IgG, IgM, IgA, and C3 perifollicularly and at the dermoepidermal junction.

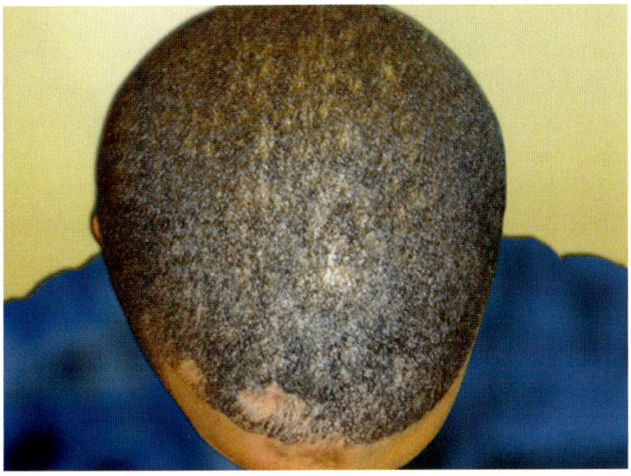

Fig. 8.5: Hyperpigmented plaques with scarring alopecia on the scalp consistent with discoid lupus erythematosus.

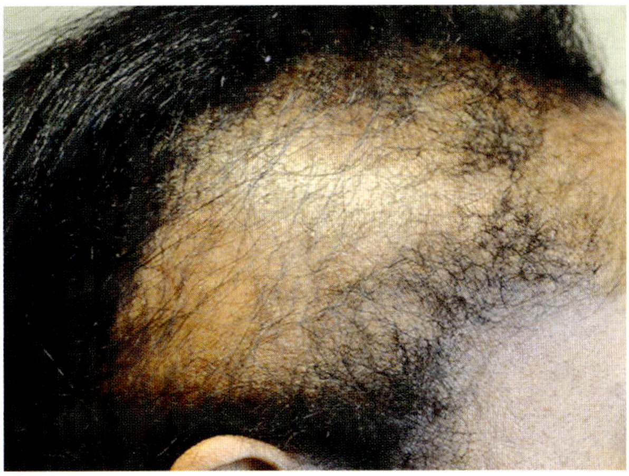

Fig. 8.6: Photograph demonstrating the "fringe sign" in a woman with traction alopecia.

Pseudopalade of Brocq

Pseudopalade of Brocq lacks an inflammatory stage and is thought to represent the late-stage cicatricial alopecia. Moreover, this clinical pattern can be observed in the end stages of LPP, CCCA, and LE. Examination can reveal ovoid, ivory, atrophic patches of scarring hair loss mainly distributed over the vertex scalp. The "footprints in snow" appearance is created by the smaller macular areas coalescing into larger plaques. A wedge-shaped scar with variable loss of elastic tissue in the upper dermis can be demonstrated on histologic examination.

Traction Alopecia (Further Discussed in HT in Blacks Chapter 9)

Termed a "biphasic alopecia," in its early stages, traction alopecia is considered nonscarring; however, prolonged involvement can lead to permanent hair loss. This entity can develop in any individual who wears tight hairstyles such as ponytails, braids, weaves, extensions, wigs, curlers, dreadlocks, or turbans; however, it is most commonly detected in black women. Any tenderness or pain associated with a hairstyle increases the risk for developing traction alopecia. If treatment is sought early and the traumatic hairstyle is ceased, hair regrowth remains possible. However, continued tension on the hair follicles will head to permanent hair loss. A diagnostic clue to early traction alopecia is shortened hairs along the temporal hairline. Continuation of the traumatic hairstyle, eventually, leads to relative preservation of the frontotemporal hairline with thinning, patches of hair loss immediately posterior to the hairline, referred to as the "fringe sign" (Fig. 8.6). Variably inflammatory, traction alopecia may also demonstrate erythematous, perifollicular scaly papules.

Histopathologic examination may mimic trichotillomania in early stages. Late-stage traction alopecia demonstrates a marked reduction in terminal hairs with the follicular epithelium replaced by columns of connective tissues.

NEUTROPHILIC PERIFOLLICULAR INFILTRATES

Folliculitis Decalvans

Folliculitis decalvans is an inflammatory, cicatricial alopecia that predominantly affects black males. Affected individuals can experience successive crops of tender, crusted, oozing pustules accompanied with the hair loss. The affected areas can become secondarily infected with *Staphylococci*; however, some argue that this entity may truly represent a primary staphylococcal infection of the scalp.

Histologic examination reveals mixed neutrophilic and granulomatous perifollicular inflammatory infiltrates in the upper portions of the follicle, with variable destruction of the follicle and sebaceous glands. End stages can demonstrate premature desquamation of the inner root sheath, destruction of the pilosebaceous unit, perifollicular fibrosis, and elastic tissue loss. Gram-positive bacteria may be seen with Gram staining.

Dissecting Cellulitis

Dissecting cellulitis can become a cosmetically disfiguring and debilitating condition. Clinical examination reveals tender, oozy, boggy, suppurative sinuses with overlying hair loss (Fig. 8.7). As part of the "follicular occlusion tetrad", individuals affected by dissecting cellulitis may also suffer with acne conglobata, hidradenitis suppurativa, and/or pilonidal cyst. Folliculitis decalvans may also be associated with this entity.

Because of its distinct features, the diagnosis of dissecting cellulitis can typically be made on clinical evaluation. However, if a biopsy is performed, histopathologic examination resembles granulation tissue with dense, neutrophilic perifollicular inflammation, and vascular proliferation in the deep dermis. In later stages, follicular destruction and perifollicular fibrosis can develop.

MIXED NEUTROPHILIC AND LYMPHOCYTIC PERIFOLLICULAR INFLAMMATION

Acne Keloidalis Nuchae

Acne keloidalis is most commonly experienced in black males or females who wear shorter hairstyles. This condition often begins with a folliculitis along the occipital scalp, likely caused by short hairs curling back into the skin and initiating a foreign-body response. Affected individuals initially demonstrate variable tender, erythematous to hyperpigmented, raised perifollicular papules along the occipital scalp. Over time, the papules may coalesce and form keloidal nodules with overlying hair loss.

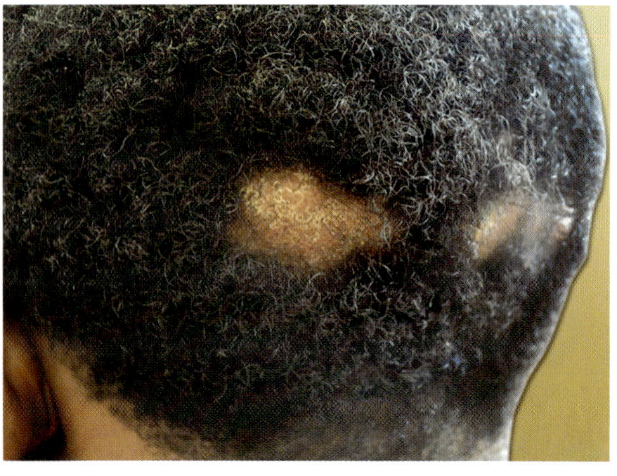

Fig. 8.7: Boggy, suppurative plaques on the occipital scalp consistent with dissecting cellulitis.

Acne keloidalis has a distinct clinical presentation; however, if histopathologic examination is obtained, it would reveal acute and chronic, variably neutrophilic, and/or mixed lymphohistiocytic perifollicular inflammatory infiltrates. Dermal scarring, follicular destruction, and concentric perifollicular lamellar fibroplasia may also be demonstrated.

SECONDARY CICATRICIAL ALOPECIAS

Secondary cicatricial alopecias occur when there is disease activity or trauma on the scalp, and the hair follicle is not the inflammatory target, but simply an "innocent bystander" (Table 8.4).

POSTSURGICAL ALOPECIA

Postsurgical alopecia is any postoperative hair loss overlying the surgical scars. Individuals who have undergone face or brow lift or scalp surgery may seek hair transplantation consultation to help camouflage these scars (Figs. 8.8A and B).

Pressure-induced (Postoperative) Alopecia

Pressure-induced alopecia is thought to be due to pressure-induced ischemia. It can occur in individuals with pressure on the scalp for a longer period during general anesthesia or in chronically ill individuals with persistent pressure on one area of the scalp.

Histology can demonstrate thrombosis, and dermal and subcutaneous perivascular inflammation in the early stages. If severe, epidermal and perieccrine necrosis, and a telogen shift occur.

Tinea Capitis

Tinea capitis is a dermatophyte infection of the hair shaft, commonly caused by *Trichophyton tonsurans*

Table 8.4: Examples of secondary cicatricial alopecias.

Trauma	*Infection*	*Postinflammatory*	*Neoplastic*
Pressure induced	Tinea capitis	Sarcoid	Basal cell carcinoma
Postsurgical scars		Morphea	Squamous cell carcinoma
Burns		Graft-versus-host disease	Alopecia neoplastica
Radiation			

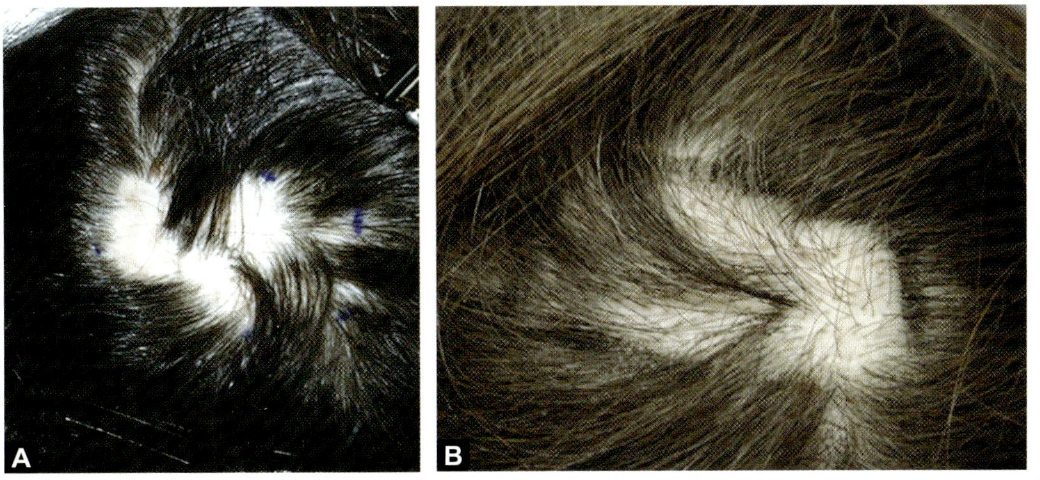

Figs. 8.8A and B: (A) A 14-year-old female with patch of scarring alopecia in the vertex scalp due to tinea capitis. (B) Modest coverage after one session of 150 follicular unit grafts into the scarred areas.

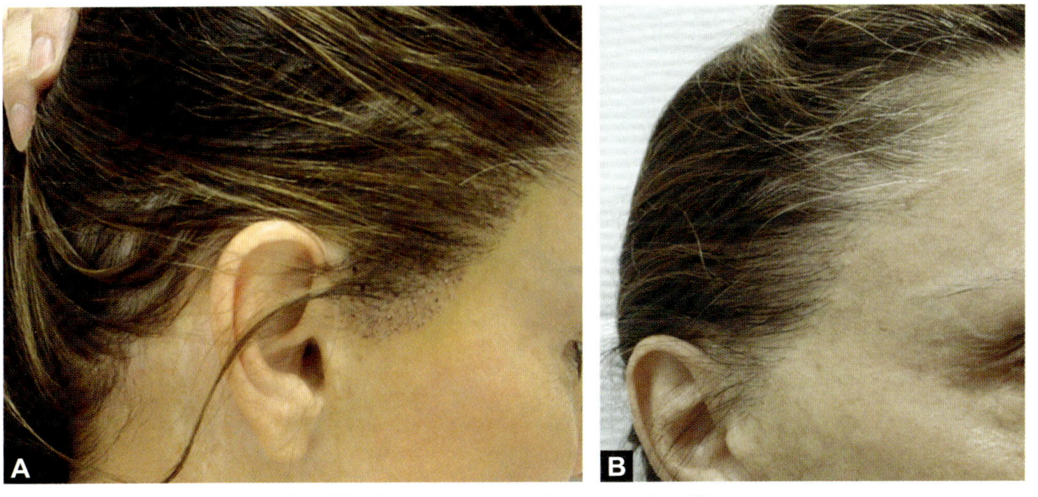

Figs. 8.9A and B: Restoration of the preauricular hairline in a woman who had undergone face-lift surgery.

and *Microsporum canis* in the United States. It most often occurs in black children or their caregivers. Careful examination reveals annular, scaly, crusted patch(es) of alopecia with variable ipsilateral occipital lymphadenitis. A chronic infection can lead to permanent scarring hair loss in the affected area (Figs. 8.9A and B). Diagnosis can be made confirmed with KOH and/or fungal culture. The involved hair follicles can reveal hyphal elements adjacent to the hair shaft (ectothrix) or within the hair shaft (endothrix).

TECHNICAL CONSIDERATIONS FOR HAIR TRANSPLANTATION IN CICATRICIAL ALOPECIA

Ultimately, when transplanting into scarring alopecias, the same general principles apply, including the anesthesia, instrumentation, graft creation, and postoperative management. With scarring alopecia, the main differences with transplantation tend to be with candidate selection, donor harvesting, recipient site creation, the total number of surgeries performed, and the management of patients' expectations (Table 8.5).

Candidate selection is of the utmost importance with respect to hair transplantation. To determine if an individual with scarring alopecia is a proper candidate, special considerations should be made. As with any patient seeking hair transplant consultation, a detailed history and scalp examination should be performed to determine the type of alopecia, donor supply, density, and caliber of the hair. Recipient areas with scarring alopecia often have decreased

Table 8.5: Differences between performing hair transplantation in scarring alopecia versus nonscarring alopecia.

	Scarring alopecia	*Nonscarring alopecia*
Number of sessions	Consider test area, then 2–4 sessions	1–2 sessions
Donor area	More unpredictable	More predictable safe donor area
Recipient area	Disease must be inactive for at least 1–2 years	May have ongoing disease activity
	Transplant with lower densities due to altered vascular supply and fibrotic tissue	Can transplant at higher densities
Outcomes	Decreased graft survival	Most grafts survive and grow
	Less coverage can be achieved with each surgery	More coverage can be achieved with greater cosmetic satisfaction

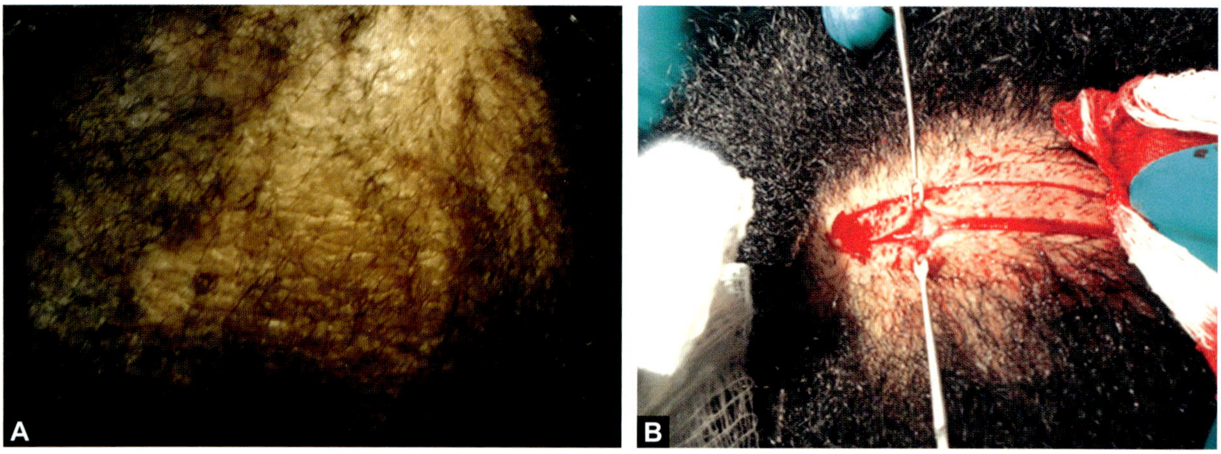

Figs. 8.10A and B: (A) An African–American female with diffuse scarring alopecia due to central centrifugal cicatricial alopecia. Example demonstrating extension of scarring alopecia into occipital donor area (B) and diminished density in the donor area due to the involvement of scarring alopecia.

blood supply and thickened fibrotic tissue, which can lead to decreased graft survival. Therefore, preoperatively, scalp thickness and available blood supply should be determined as best can be achieved.

With primary cicatricial alopecias, hair transplantation should only be considered if the involved areas have been inactive for 1-2 years. The condition should be quiescent with no anticipation of further disease activity. This decreases the risk of targeted inflammation of the transplanted hairs and likelihood of disease flare. A postoperative biopsy may be warranted to evaluate for disease reactivation, if graft survival is less than expected or with any signs of inflammation.

DONOR AREA

The optimal area to harvest donor grafts is the horizontal zone in the midoccipital scalp with hair transplantation for the treatment of androgenetic alopecia. This is considered the "safe zone" where disease activity is less likely. Because androgenetic alopecia is a progressive condition, harvesting from the "safe zone" should prevent a visible donor scar. In addition, due to the theory of donor dominance, these grafts are uninvolved from disease activity and, theoretically, should grow indefinitely. Comparatively, with scarring alopecia, disease activity may have involved the "safe zone". Therefore, on preoperative evaluation, it is important to determine where viable grafts can be harvested from and whether the patient has adequate donor supply to produce a desirable cosmetic outcome (Figs. 8.10A and B).

Donor density may be even more limited in individuals affected by scarring alopecia; therefore, it is a major determinant of the success and overall cosmetic effect of the procedure. Density is determined by follicular units per square centimeter in contrast to the number of hairs per square centimeter. Typically, the goal is to place at least 20–40 follicular unit grafts per square centimeter. However, with cicatricial alopecia, less may be acceptable due to decreased density.

Table 8.6: Factors to consider when determining donor harvesting method.

	Strip	*Follicular unit extraction*
Duration of surgery	Considerably shorter time to harvest	Longer harvesting time
	Potentially longer time to trim grafts	Less time to trim grafts
	Same time for planting grafts	Same time for planting grafts
Number of grafts	Typically more grafts can be harvested in the defined safe harvesting zone	Less grafts harvested, may need more than one session
Overall cosmetic outcome	Same	Same
Considerations for scarring alopecia	Because of unpredictable donor area, may have more variable density in the linear area	Can choose areas of higher density and areas not involved with alopecia for harvesting
Scar	Visible linear scar	No visible linear scar, may see hypopigmented dots or risk moth-eaten look with over harvesting

When transplanting into scarring alopecia, hair caliber may become even more crucial. Because of reduced vascular supply, grafts should be transplanted at lower densities; curlier, larger-caliber hairs will achieve greater cover than individuals with straight, finer caliber hairs.

DONOR HARVESTING

There are two methods of donor harvesting: (1) strip excision and (2) follicular unit extraction (FUE). There are several factors to consider when determining which method to use, including patient preference (Table 8.6).

Typically with strip excision, the surgeon can harvest more grafts at a quicker rate with decreased transection. However, there is a visible linear scar present. Therefore, the strip excision is advised for individuals with longer occipital hair and those who require more grafts. In addition, because large areas typically need to be shaved in the donor region, FUE may be less preferable to women. Follicular unit extraction may also be more technically difficult in individuals with very curly hair.

One of the main advantages of choosing the FUE may produce scattered, hypopigmented, macular scars and diffuse, moth-like thinning of the occipital region. However, in patients with scarring alopecia, FUE is recommended for individuals where a linear scar in the occiput would be visible, those with limited donor supply, when less grafts are required, and those who have a tendency to develop widened, hypertrophic scars.

RECIPIENT AREA

Vascular Supply

A major limitation of transplantation into scar tissue can be decreased vascular supply compared to normal tissue, leading to poor graft survival. Several small incisions with an 18-gauge needle can be placed to assess prior to transplantation. Dense packing with increased grafts per square centimeter is not advised due to the poor blood supply and subsequent risk of ischemic necrosis. Alternatively, a test area may be performed with lower densities. In addition, an application of 2–5% minoxidil preoperatively or pentoxyphylline 400 mg, 2 weeks preoperatively, may increase available blood supply.

SCALP THICKNESS AND FIBROSIS

Thickness and texture of scalps with scarring alopecia are greatly variable; however, scars can be hypertrophic or atrophic. The skin may be tough, tacked down, inelastic, and/or friable. Deeper incision in hypertrophic, thicker scars may be considered to reach the vascular supply. With atrophic scars, to compensate for the lack of subcutaneous tissue to support the follicular graft, incisions should be made at a more acute angle.

OTHER CONSIDERATIONS

Other technical considerations can be made when performing hair transplantation into scarring alopecia. A small test area may need to be performed in patients who may be at risk for decreased graft

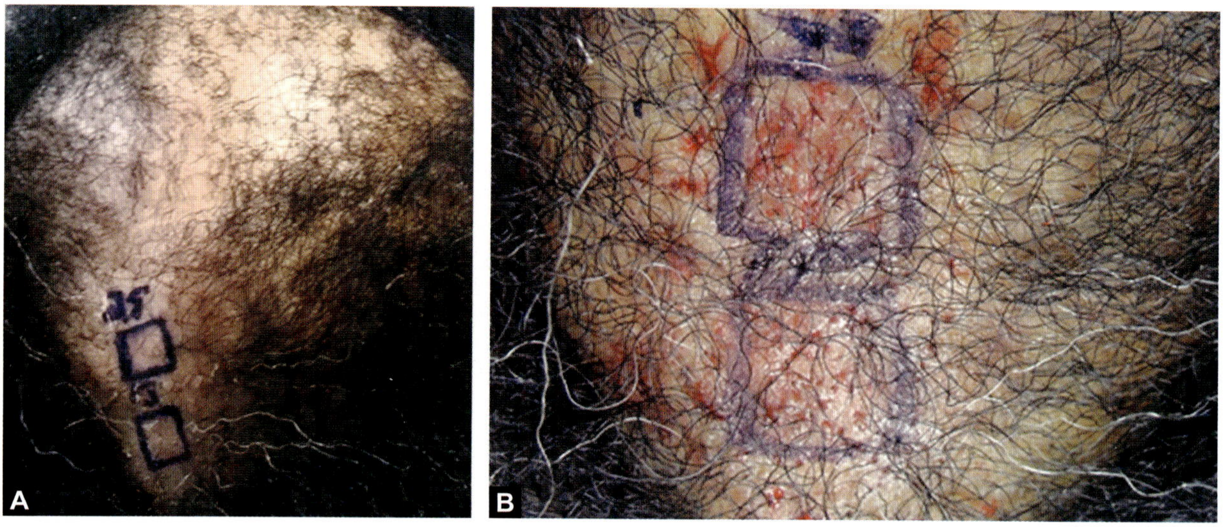

Figs. 8.11A and B: (A) Diffuse scarring alopecia due to central centrifugal cicatricial alopecia. Photographs demonstrating two 1 cm^2 test areas with 15 grafts per square centimeter and 25 grafts per square centimeter, (B) immediately after transplantation into test areas.

Table 8.7: Summary of the technical considerations to treat cicatricial alopecia.
If caused by inflammatory alopecia, disease should be inactive without progression and inactive on biopsy for 1–2 years.
Consider starting with a test area with decreased density.
Perform smaller, less dense sessions every 9–12 months.
Consider minoxidil or pentoxyphylline to improve blood flow.
Consider making incisions at an acute angle.

survival, based on preoperatively evaluation. Initially, a 1-2 cm^2 area can be transplanted (Figs. 8.11A and B). After 9-12 months, if graft survival is assessed to be adequate, a larger session can be performed.

Transplanting at decreased densities is advised with scarring alopecia (10-30 follicular units/cm^2) compared to androgenetic alopecia (at least 20-40 follicular units/cm^2). In addition, the patient is counseled that additional sessions may need to be performed every 9-12 months, each time achieving higher densities.

Overall, when performing hair transplantation into scarring alopecia, setting expectations is pertinent. Patients must be aware of the potential for decreased graft survival with the inability to transplant at higher densities. Therefore, full coverage may not be achieved, and 2-4 sessions may be necessary. In addition, because of the fibrotic tissue in the recipient area, initially, the hairs may grow in kinky and then straighten with additional hair cycles. Patients who can accept the potential limitations of the procedure are generally content with any cosmetic improvement. Therefore, any patient with end-stage cicatricial alopecia, in particular, can be offered hair transplantation as an option for the treatment of their cosmetically disfiguring conditions (Table 8.7).

BIBLIOGRAPHY

1. Alvarez MS, Silverberg, NB. Tinea Capitis. Cutis. 2006;78(3):189-96.
2. Avram MR, Rogers NE. Hair Transplantation. New York, NY: Cambridge University Press; 2010.
3. Borovicka JH, Thomas L, Prince C, et al. Scarring alopecia: clinical and pathologic study of 54 African-American women. Int J Dermatol. 2009;48(8):840-5.
4. Callender VD, McMichael AJ, Cohen GF. Medical and surgical therapies for alopecias in black women. Dermatol Ther. 2004;17(2):164-76.
5. Hordinsky M. Cicatricial alopecia: discoid lupus erythematosus. Dermatol Ther. 2008;21:245-8.
6. Kang H, Alzolibani AA, Otberg, N. Lichen planopilaris. Dermatol Ther. 2008;21:249-56.
7. McElwee KJ. Etiology of cicatriciai alopecias: a basic science point of view. Dermatol Ther. 2008;21:212-20.
8. Mehregan DA, Van Hale HM, Muller, SA. Lichen planopilaris: clinical and pathologic study of forty-five patients. J Am Acad Dermatol. 1992;27:935-42.
9. Olson EA, Bergfeld WF, Costerelis G, et al. Summary of North American Hair Research Society (NAHRS)-sponsored Workshop on Cicatricial Alopecia, Duke University Medical Center. J Am Acad Dermatol. 2003;48:103-10.
10. Rongioletti F, Christana K. Cicatricial (scarring) alopecias: an overview of pathogenesis, classification, diagnosis, and trreatment. Am J Clin Dermatol. 2012;13(4):247-60.

11. Rose PT, Shapiro R. Transplanting into scar tissue and areas of cicatricial alopecia. In: Shapiro R, Unger W (Eds). Hair Transplantation. New York: Marcel Dekker; 2004. pp. 606-10.
12. Ross EK, Tan E, Shapiro J. Update on primary cicatricial alopecias. J Am Acad Dermatol. 2005;53: 1-37.
13. Somani N, Bergfeld WF. Cicatricial alopecia: classification and histopathology. Dermatol Ther. 2008; 21:221-47.
14. Sperling LC, Cowper SE. The histopathology of primary cicatricial alopecia. Semin Cutan Med Surg. 2006;25:41-50.
15. Tan KT, Messenger AG. Frontal fibrosing alopecia: clinical presentations and prognosis. Br J Dermatol. 2009;160:75-9.
16. Unger W, Unger R, Wesley C. The surgical treatment of cicatricial alopecia. Dermatol Ther. 2008; 21(4):295-311.
17. Viglizzo G, Verrini AM, Rongioletti F. Familial Lassueur–Graham–Little–Piccardi syndrome. Dermatology. 2004;208:142-4.
18. Whiting DA, Olson EA. Central centrifugal cicatricial alopecia. Dermatol Ther. 2008;21:268-78.
19. Wiles JC, Hansen RC. Postoperative (pressure) alopecia. J Am Acad Dermatol. 1985;12(Pts): 195-8.

CHAPTER

9

Hair Transplantation in Blacks

Duane Dilworth, Meena K Singh

INTRODUCTION

Hair transplantation provides both men and women a permanent solution for hair loss. According to the International Society of Hair Restoration Surgery Practice Census, 88,304 hair transplantations were performed in the United States in 2012.[1] Although there is minimal data detailing the racial background of these patients, it is presumed that more black patients are seeking hair restoration surgery as the demographics of the United States change.

Hair transplantation was pioneered by Dr Norman Orentreich and Dr Shoji Okuda in mid 1900s, using 4-mm punch autografting from the occipital scalp.[2] This method of hair transplantation often resulted in large "plugs" that appeared unnatural and unsightly. Additionally, early studies found a discrepancy in the success rate of hair transplantation in blacks.[3] These studies outlined variations in techniques based on the curliness of the hair follicle. Advances in hair transplant, by Bernstein et al. in the 1990s lead to discovery of follicular unit transplantation (FUT).[4] This modality of hair transplantation has been shown to lead to higher success rates in hair transplantation, while providing a more natural appearance. Due to variations in donor density and caliber, types of alopecia, and potential complications, FUT in blacks warrants special technical considerations.

CANDIDATE SELECTION

With potential hair transplant recipients, candidate selection is important. Most black male patients seek consultation for hair transplant to treat androgenetic alopecia. Black females typically desire hair transplantation to treat traction alopecia (TA) and/or endstage central centrifugal cicatricial alopecia (CCCA). Proper diagnosis of the type of hair loss is imperative. This entails a detailed history, scalp examination, and often histologic examination. In addition, proper treatment of the underlying mechanism of hair loss is imperative to the overall success of hair restoration surgery.

Traction alopecia is a common form of hair loss among blacks arising from long-term use of braids, ponytails, hair weaves, and other styling techniques (Figs. 9.1 and 9.2). The distribution of hair loss in TA tends to be, but not limited to, the bitemporal regions, frontal hairline, and occiput. Traction alopecia is classified as a nonscarring alopecia and is generally reversible in its early stages. Patients should be counseled onappropriate styling techniques that minimize traction. Medical therapies include topical minoxidil and intralesional corticosteroids.

Central centrifugal cicatricial alopecia (discussed in further detail in Scarring Alopecia chapter) is an inflammatory, scarring alopecia commonly seen in black women. Early stages of this disease are characterized by central hair breakage, perifollicular hyperkeratosis, erythema, and thinning at the vertex of the scalp. Later stages of this disease process are marked by centrifugal clearing of the involved area.[5] The pathogenesis of this disease is not fully elucidated, but is related to chemical relaxers and traumatic

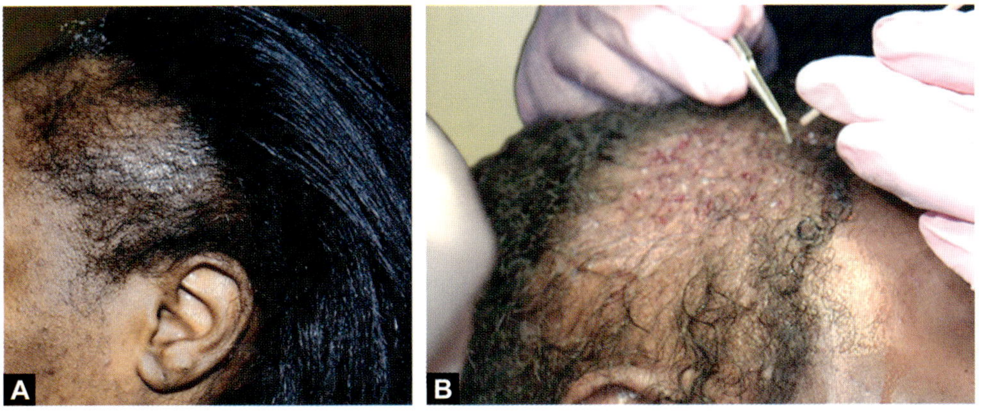

Figs. 9.1A and B: (A) Preoperative photo demonstrating an African-American woman with traction alopecia; (B) Placing grafts intraoperatively.

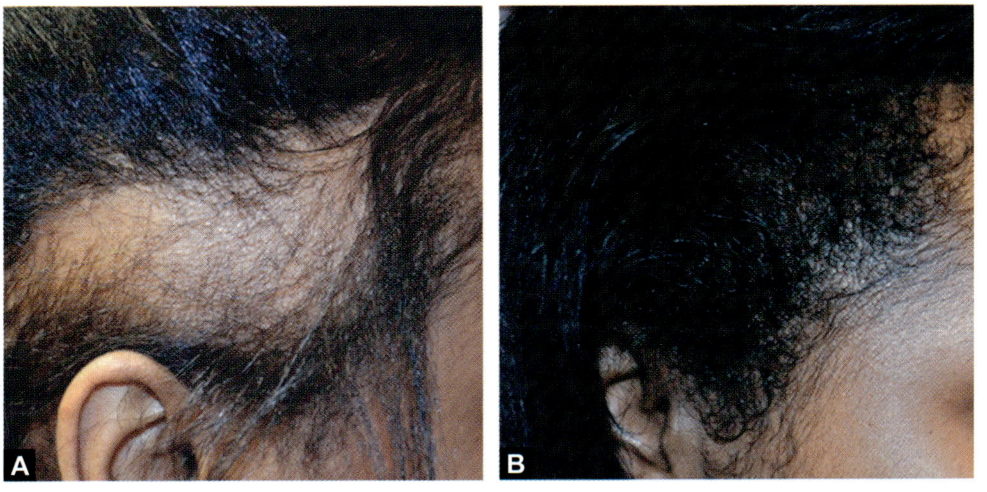

Figs. 9.2A and B: A black female with traction alopecia. (A) Preoperative photo; (B) After hair transplantation.
Courtesy: Dr. Nicole Rogers.

hairstyling practices. Prior to hair transplantation, it is important to ensure the recipient site is not actively inflamed.

Proper medical treatment is required prior to hair transplantation in order to achieve the best results. Most physicians utilize medical management for a minimum of 9–12 months to suppress ongoing inflammation that could be detrimental to newly transplanted grafts. Current medical treatment options for CCCA are tailored to controlling the inflammatory process with topical and intralesional corticosteroids, immunosuppresants, and anti-inflammatory agents (Figs. 9.3 and 9.4).

Keloids and hypertrophic scars should always be a concern when a patient has a positive personal or familial history. Very few incidences of scalp keloids after hair transplantation have been documented. However, the incidence of keloid formation in highly pigmented skin types is 4.5–16%.[6] Additionally, darker pigmented skin types are 15 times more likely to develop keloids than less pigmented skin types.[7]

Differences in Hair Characteristics (Table 9.1)

When assessing black patients for hair transplantation, it is important to consider the differences in hair morphology between various races. Understanding these distinct differences can result in an increase in successful follicular unit harvesting and transplantation. Black hair is typically tightly curled, c-shaped, spiral, or helical, with a curved follicle, and a flattened, elliptical shape in cross section (Figs. 9.5 and 9.6). Under light microscopy, it contains multiple knots and breaks along the hair shaft.

Blacks generally have a significantly lower hair density in comparison to whites. In a retrospective case series, blacks were found to have 21.4 total

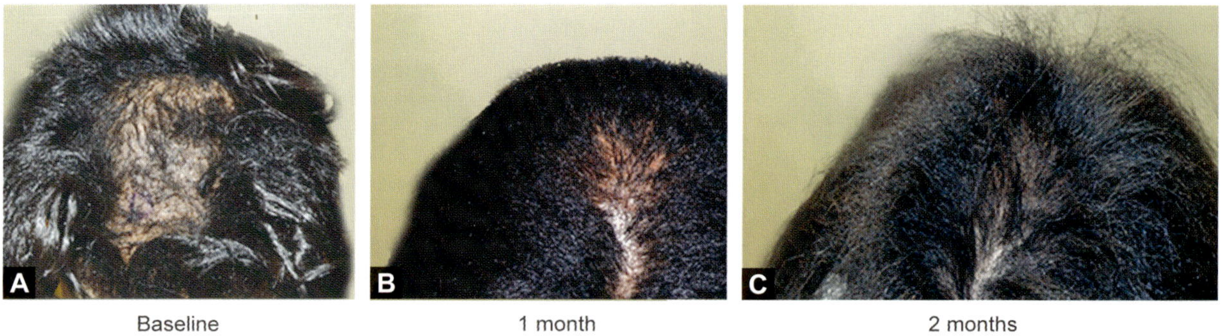

Figs. 9.3A to C: A young African-American woman with biopsy proven CCCA with moderate lymphohistiocytic perifollicular inflammation. (A) Scarring hairloss over the vertex scalp; (B) Marked improvement, one month after treatment with intralesional triamcinolone, minoxidil, and doxycycline; (C) Seeing significant improvement, two months after treatment was initiated.

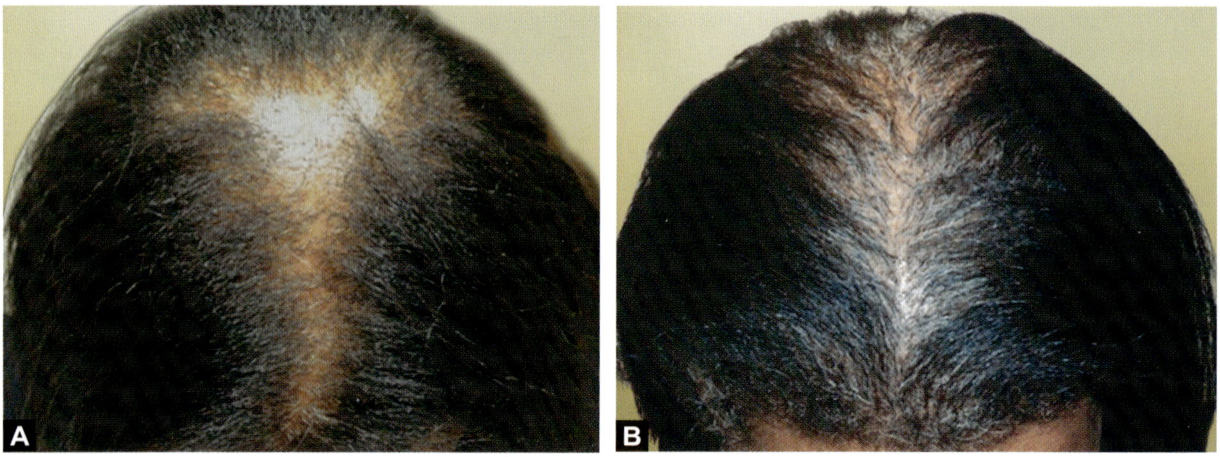

Figs. 9.4A and B: (A) Preoperative photo of an African-American woman with CCCA; (B) Significant improvement seen after hair transplantation. *Courtesy*: Dr. Nicole Rogers.

Table 9.1: Illustrating the differences in hair characteristics in blacks compared to Caucasians.

Hair Characteristic	*Blacks*	*Caucasians*
Shape	Curly	Wavy/Straight
Cross section	Elliptical	Oval
Follicular units per square centimeter	60	100

follicles from a 4-mm punch biopsy while Caucasians had 35.5 total follicles.[8] Blacks were also found to have fewer terminal follicles when compared to whites (18.4 vs 30.4) and decreased anagen hairs (17.3 vs 28.8).[9] Although the density is lower in blacks, the curlier hair provides better coverage. In addition, there is less contrast between hair color and scalp color.[10] Therefore, surgeons should be less deterred in blacks with lower donor supply.

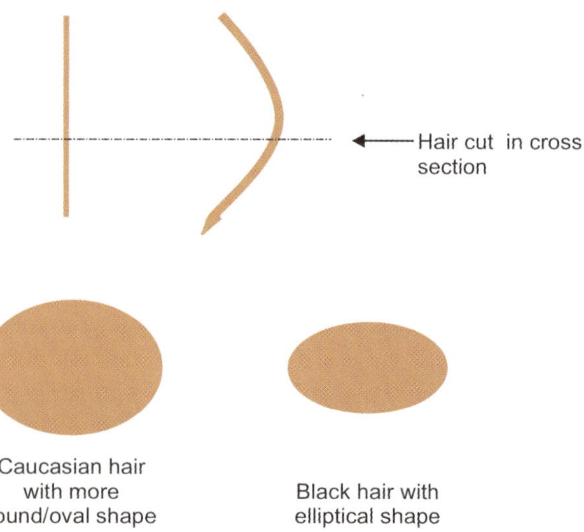

Fig. 9.5: Cross-sectional analysis of Caucasian hair (more round and ovoid) compared to black hair (elliptical).

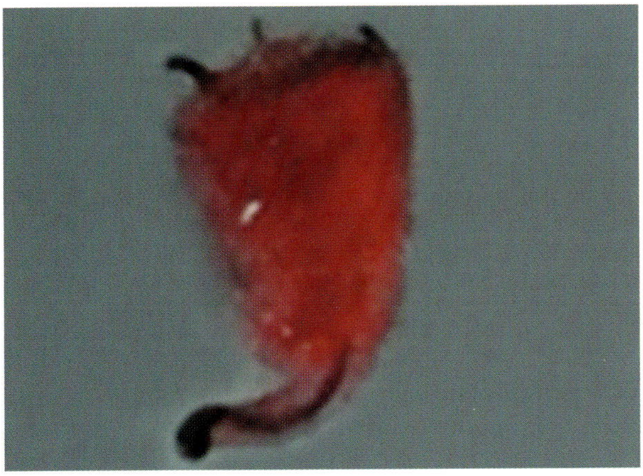

Fig. 9.6: Demonstrating the "C-shaped" subcutaneous course of the hair follicle in blacks.

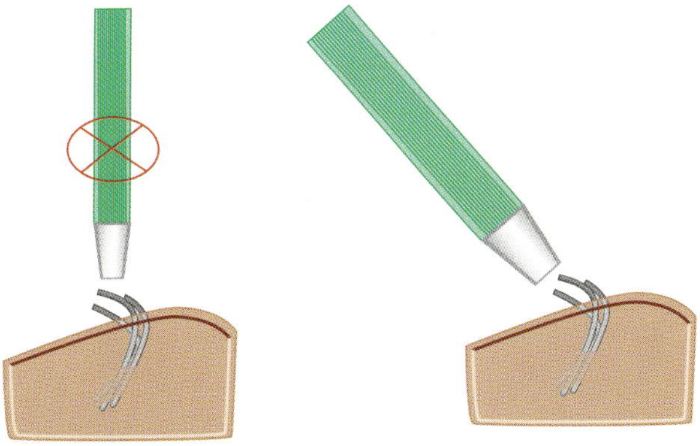

Fig. 9.7: Demonstrating the need for an acute angle of entry and a larger diameter punch tool in curly hair.
Source: Photo adapted from "Technical considerations of FUE in African-Americans," Singh M.K. and Avram MR, Dermatol Surg 2013.

DONOR AREA

The curvature of the hair follicle in black patients increases the rate of transection. Studies using flexible blades, generally used in shave biopsies, have proven to be beneficial in decreasing transection rates. The flexibility of the blade allows the operator to bend the blade easily to match the curvature of the hair follicle. Strip excision is favorable in patients with longer hair lengths, which tend to hide the linear scar. This procedure is generally carried out by a single 10- or 15-blade scalpel. A double-bladed scalpel is less favorable in black patients secondary to an increased risk of transecting donor follicles.[11,12]

In black males that wear shorter hairstyles, follicular unit extraction (FUE) is the preferred method of hair transplant surgery. Strip harvesting is less favorable due to scar visibility with low-cropped hair. Follicular unit extraction utilizes multiple 1-mm punch excisions to obtain follicular units. Major drawbacks in this technique include increased follicular transection when compared to strip harvesting and increased donor harvesting time. Using punch excisions >1 mm has been proven to decrease transection of the hair follicles in black patients; however, larger-diameter punches increase the risk of hypopigmented macular scars.[13] With tightly curled hair, angling the punch instrument parallel to the angle of the exiting hair will improve donor harvesting. Manual punch tools may have an additional advantage over motorized punch tools (Fig. 9.7).

HAIRLINE DESIGN

The hairline is a primary determinant of the face shape and a youthful appearance. Most patients seeking hair restoration surgery hope to regain their hairline prior to hair loss. Therefore, the hairline design often defines the success of hair transplantation. Planning the hairline involves creating a natural appearing hairline with an appropriate amount of hair density.

The same general principles of hairline design apply to black males. Smaller follicular unit grafts should be used. However, a flatter, straight hairline is more desirable and can look natural in blacks (Figs. 9.8 and 9.9). When creating a frontal hairline in black men, the physician must counsel patients about the design that will appear the most natural years after transplantation. In addition to the hair loss at the time of presentation, the patient must be informed of continued hairline recession and thinning over time. Optimal results are achieved by balancing the frontal hairline with the temporal and posterior hairlines.

KEY CONCEPTS FOR HAIR TRANSPLANTATION IN BLACKS

- Proper diagnosis is important for hair transplantation.
- Black males typically seek treatment for male pattern hair loss (MPHL).
- Black females typically seek treatment for TA and/or CCCA.

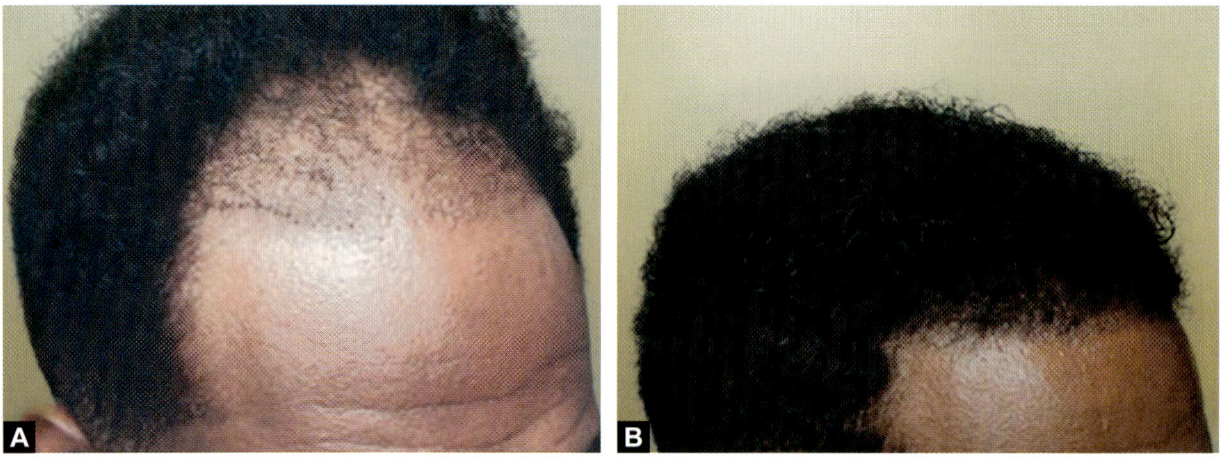

Figs. 9.8A and B: (A) Preoperative photo of an African-American male with Norwood Class III male pattern hair loss; (B) Demonstrating a straighter hairline design, suitable for black males. Courtesy: Denise Kernan.

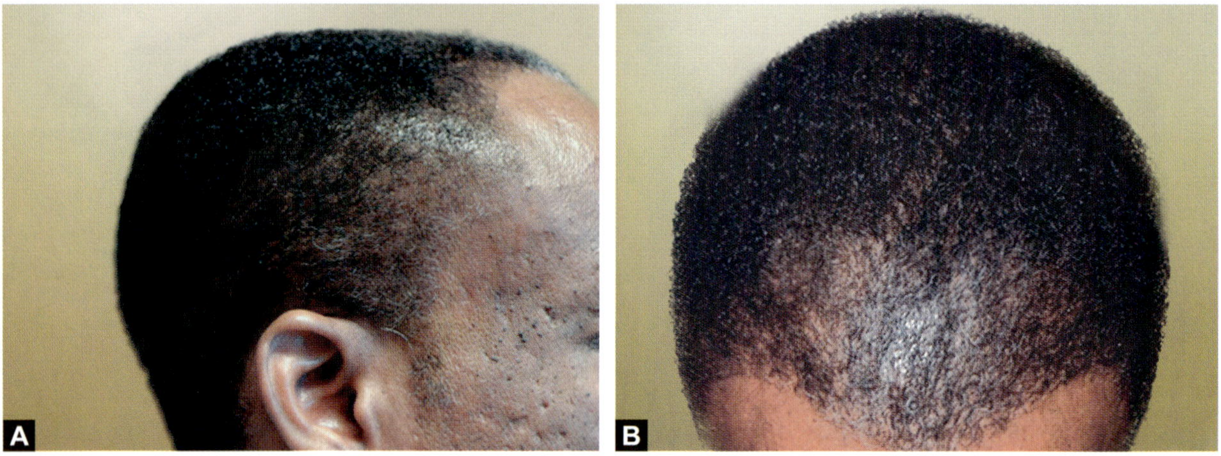

Figs. 9.9A and B: Postoperative photo after hair transplantation performed by another surgeon. The patient's hairline was given a more Caucasian, recessed hairline, which appears unnatural.

- Any active inflammation should be managed medically before hair transplant can be considered.
- Black hair is coiled and forms a "C shape" under the skin.
- Although blacks have less density, the curlier hairs and decreased contrast between hair color and skin color, provide better coverage.
- With strip excision, graft creation is more difficult. A curved blade is recommended for graft dissection.
- With FUE, transection rates can be higher in curly hair. Therefore, a larger punch is recommended.
- Hairline design can be flatter and straighter in black males.

REFERENCES

1. International Society of Hair Restoration Surgery. (2013). Practice Census. [online]. Available from http://www.ishrs.org/statistics-research.htm [Accessed December, 2014].
2. Pierce HE. The uniqueness of hair transplantation in black patients. J Natl Med Assoc. 1976;68(4):343.
3. Selmanowitz VJ, Orentreich N. Hair transplantation in blacks. J Natl Med Assoc. 1973;65(6):471-82.
4. Bernstein RM, Rassman WR, Szaniawski W, et al. Follicular transplantation. Int J Aesthetic Restorative Surg. 1995;3:119–32.
5. Ogunleye T, McMichael AJ, Olsen EA. Central centrifugal cicatricial alopecia: what has been achieved, current clues for future research. Dermatol Clin. 2014;32(2):173-8.

6. Rockwell WB, Cohen IK, Ehrilich HP. Keloids and hypertrophic scars: a comprehensive review. Plast Reconstr Surg. 1989;84:827-37.
7. Alhady SM, Sivanantharajah K. Keloids in various races. A review of 175 cases. Plast Reconstr Surg. 1969;44(6):564-6.
8. Sperling LC. Hair density in African Americans. Arch Dermatol. 1999;135(6):656-8.
9. Vernall DG. Study of the size and shape of hair from four races of men. Am J Phys Anthropol. 1961;19:345.
10. Khumalo NP, Doe PT, Dawber RP, et al. What is normal black African hair? A light and scanning electron-microscopic study. J Am Acad Dermatol. 2000;43(5 Pt 1):814-20.
11. Epstein J, Bared A, Kuka G. Ethnic considerations in hair restoration surgery. Facial Plast Surg Clin North Am. 2014;22(3):427-37.
12. Lam SM, Karamanovski E. Hair restoration in the ethnic patient and review of hair transplant fundamentals. Facial Plast Surg Clin North Am. 2010;18 (1):35-42.
13. Singh MK, Avram MR. Technical considerations for follicular unit extraction in African-American Hair. Dermatol Surg. 2013;39(8):1282-4.

CHAPTER

10

Medications Used in Hair Transplantation

Duane Dilworth, Meena K Singh

INTRODUCTION

Hair transplantation is a successful method to enhance and restore areas of hair loss. It does not, however, address progressive thinning in the affected areas. The final cosmetic outcome is a result of the number of grafts transplanted minus ongoing hair loss. Therefore, controlling the ongoing hair loss with medication is recommended.

To date, there are only two medications approved by the Food and Drug Administration (FDA) for the treatment of hair loss. These medications include minoxidil (Rogaine) and finasteride (Propecia). Additionally, antiandrogens have shown to have some efficacy in hair growth, but are not currently FDA approved for the sole treatment of hair loss. It is important to understand the proper use of these medications when treating patients with alopecia. When these medications are used as an adjuvant to hair transplantation, there is an increase in overall hair density, a decreased risk of postoperative telogen effluvium, and decreased duration for graft growth.

MINOXIDIL

Topical minoxidil (Rogaine) is the most commonly used agent for the treatment of hair loss. In 1988 and 1991, the FDA approved a 2% minoxidil topical solution for the treatment of male pattern hair loss (MPHL) and female androgenetic alopecia, respectively. Later in 1997, a 5% minoxidil topical solution was FDA approved for male androgenetic alopecia. Most recently, a 5% minoxidil foam became available in 2006.

Minoxidil was initially developed as an oral antihypertensive medication, working as a direct vasodilator to decrease systemic resistance and decrease blood pressure.[1] Patients prescribed with oral minoxidil were observed to have hypertrichosis as an adverse side effect. The exact mechanism of action for the cause of secondary hypertrichosis is not yet understood. It is presumed that minoxidil causes prolongation of the anagen phase of the hair cycle and an increase in the hair follicle size. Minoxidil was proven to rethicken hair diameter and stop the progression of hair loss in 85–90% of patients.[2] Complete effects are typically observed approximately 6–9 months after the initiation of this therapy. In addition, minoxidil may decrease the risk of postoperative telogen effluvium and increase graft survival and growth.[3]

The 5% formulation is recommended over the 2% formulation. In a 24-week randomized, single-blind trial of 5% minoxidil foam once daily versus 2% minoxidil solution twice daily, the 5% foam showed noninferior target hair count and target area hair width. Additionally, there was a significant decrease in local pruritus and dandruff.[4]

FINASTERIDE

Finasteride (Propecia) is a competitive and specific inhibitor of the type II isoform of 5α-reductase, the enzyme responsible for converting intracellular testosterone to 5-DHT. Type II 5α-reductase is primarily found in hair follicle, prostate, seminal vesicles, and epididymis. This isoform functions at the hair follicle by decreasing scalp and serum dihydrotestosterone (DHT), thus decreasing hair follicle miniaturization.

Finasteride was FDA approved for the treatment of MPHL in men with mild-to-moderate hair loss of scalp vertex and mid-scalp area. However, it used off label for the treatment of female pattern hair loss (FPHL), as well. Finasteride is marketed as a once a day 1 mg tablet and is now generic. Studies have shown that finasteride slows the progression of hair loss in 88–92% of patients and promotes hair regrowth in 65% of patients.[5]

This drug is typically well tolerated. However, the most common side effect encountered is sexual dysfunction, which was observed in 1–2% of the Finasteride MPHL Study Group. In a systematic review comprised of 12 randomized controlled trials to evaluate the efficacy and safety of finasteride versus placebo, finasteride increased hair count, while increasing the risk of sexual dysfunction.[6] Interestingly, the risk of discontinuing treatment because of sexual adverse effects was similar to the placebo.

In a study comparing the incidence of sexual adverse effects of finasteride 5 mg, patients informed of possible sexual side effects were found to have more sexual side effects than the group of patients who were not counseled about such side effects, 43.6% versus 17%.[7] Further studies need to be conducted to determine if finasteride leads to persistent sexual adverse effects.

DUTASTERIDE

Dutasteride (Avodart) is a medication currently marketed for the treatment of benign prostatic hyperplasia. Not only does dutasteride inhibit type II 5α-reductase, like finasteride, it also inhibits type I 5α-reductase that is predominantly found in sebaceous glands. Dutasteride 0.5 mg daily is currently used off label in the treatment of hair loss. When compared to finasteride, it is three times more potent at inhibiting type II 5α-reductase and 100 times more potent at inhibiting type I 5α-reductase.[8] In a 24-week study, dutasteride reduced serum DHT levels better than finasteride (94.7% vs. 70.8%).[9] A randomized, double-blind phase III trial showed an increase in mean hair counts when compared to placebo (12.2 cm^{-2} vs 4.7 cm^{-2}).[10] Although dutasteride is currently not FDA approved for the treatment of androgenetic alopecia, these studies show promising results that could help elucidate the value of dutasteride in hair loss.

KETOCONAZOLE

Ketoconazole (Nizarol) is a broad spectrum, imidazole antifungal that blocks fungal cytochrome P450 thus decreasing cell wall permeability. Due to its inhibitory effect on steroid biosynthesis, it has led to use in advanced prostate cancer. Prior studies have demonstrated an effective treatment for androgenetic alopecia with ketoconazole 2% shampoo. A prior study showed that when used as an adjuvant with finasteride, ketoconazole 2% can potentially further reduce DHT production in patients with androgenetic alopecia (AGA).[11-14] A recent study analyzing the promotive effect of ketoconazole 2% in mice found significant hair growth.[15] These investigators also found that nonandrogen-insensitive hair was also affected by ketoconazole, indicating its use may also be androgen independent.

SPIRONOLACTONE

Spironolactone is an aldosterone antagonist marketed for its antihypertensive and diuretic effects. This medication is FDA approved for primary hyperaldosteronism, chronic heart failure, and essential hypertension. Secondarily, it affects adrenal androgen production through blockade of androgen receptors, thus increasing testosterone clearance and estradiol production. When used in women with polycystic ovarian syndrome, women noted reduction in hirsutism.[16] Numerous studies have shown effective hair regrowth with continued treatment of spironolactone 100–200 mg daily.

PLATELET-RICH PLASMA

Platelet-rich plasma (PRP) injections are a nonsurgical treatment modality oriented toward biologic regeneration of affected hair follicles. When activated, platelets secrete a number of cytokines and growth factors that are an integral part of wound healing, such as platelet-derived growth factor, epidermal growth factor, transforming growth factor, and vascular endothelial growth factor. Because of their important function, concentrated platelet preparations have been used in damaged joints in the orthopedic field, and utilized for facial rejuvenation by cosmetic dermatologists and plastic surgeons.

Over the last 3 years, several studies have suggested that PRP promotes hair growth and increases hair density. When used as an adjunct to hair restoration surgery, grafts that were pretreated with PRP solution demonstrated better density and graft survival. Although PRP injections seem to be a promising advancement in the field of hair loss, human clinical trials have been quite limited. In a pilot study of 64 participants with androgenetic alopecia treated with PRP injections, the authors demonstrated significant clinical improvement at 6 months.[17] However,

Table 10.1: Treatment options to control ongoing hair loss.
Minoxidil 5% foam or solution daily
Ketoconazole shampoo daily
Finasteride 1 mg orally daily
Dutasteride .5 mg orally daily
Spironolactone 100–200 mg orally daily
Platelet-rich plasma injections
Low-level light laser stimulation

the pilot study had numerous limitations including platelet concentration, frequency of treatments, and long-term follow-up.

LOW-LEVEL LIGHT LASER THERAPY

Low-level light laser devices have been increasingly used not only as primary treatment of androgenetic alopecia but also as an adjunct to hair transplant. These devices typically use 600–650 nm wavelengths to cause a biostimulatory effect on hair growth. Recently, several studies have shown increased density and follicular thickness with these devices.[18-22]

In summary, there are numerous methods to control ongoing hair loss in patients who have undergone hair transplant (Table 10.1). Because the final outcome of the procedure is dependent on preventing further hair loss, patients should be encouraged to treat progressive hair loss in the recipient areas.

REFERENCES

1. Limas CJ, Fresis ED. Minoxidil in severe hypertension with renal failure. Effect of its addition to conventional antihypertensive drugs. Am J Cardiol. 1973;31:353-61.
2. Messenger AG, Rundegren J. Minoxidil: mechanisms of action on hair growth. Br J Dermatol. 2004; 150:186-94.
3. Rousso DE, Kim SW. A review of medical and surgical treatment options for androgenetic alopecia. JAMA Facial Plast Surg. 2014;16(6):444-50.
4. Blume-Peytavi U, Hillmann K, Dietz E, et al. A randomized, single-blind trial of 5% minoxidil foam once daily versus 2% minoxidil solution twice daily in the treatment of androgenetic alopecia in women. J Am Acad Dermatol. 2011;65(6):1126-34 e2.
5. Mella J, Perret M, Manzotti M, et al. Efficacy and safety of finasteride therapy for androgenetic alopecia: a systematic review. Arch Dermatol. 2010; 146(10):1141-50.
6. Irwig MS, Kolukula S. Persistent sexual side effects of finasteride for male pattern hair loss. J Sex Med. 2011;8:1747-53.
7. Mondaini N, Gontero P, Giubilei G, et al. Finasteride 5 mg and sexual side effects: how many of these are related to a nocebo phenomenon? J Sex Med. 2007;4:1708-12.
8. Clark RV, Hermann DJ, Cunningham GR, et al. Marked suppression of dihydrotestosterone in men with benign prostatic hyperplasia by dutasteride, a dual 5α-reductase inhibitor, J Clin Endocrinol Metab. 2004;89(5):2179-84.
9. Olsen EA, Hordinsky M, Whiting D, et al. The importance of dual 5α-reductase inhibition in the treatment of male pattern hair loss: results of a randomized placebo-controlled study of dutasteride versus finasteride. J Am Acad Dermatol. 2006;55: 1014-23.
10. Eun HC, Kwon OS, Yeon JH, et al. Efficacy, safety, and tolerability of dutasteride 0.5 mg once daily in male patients with male pattern hair loss: a randomized, double-blind, placebo-controlled, phase III study. J Am Acad Dermatol. 2010;63(2):252-8.
11. Hugo Perez BS. Ketocazole as an adjunct to finasteride in the treatment of androgenetic alopecia in men. Med Hypotheses. 2004;62(1):112-5.
12. Deruyne FM, Witjes FA. Ketoconazole high dose (H.D.) in the management of hormonally pretreated patients with progressive metastatic prostate cancer. Prog Clin Biol Res. 1987;243A:301-13.
13. Banka N, Bunagan K, Shapiro J. Pattern hair loss in men. J Dermatol Clin. 2013;31(1):129-40.
14. Levy LL, Emer JJ. Female pattern alopecia: current perspectives. Int J Womens Health. 2013;5:541-56.
15. Aldhalimi MA, Hadi NR, Ghafil FA. Promotive effect of topical ketoconazole, minoxidil, and minoxidil with tritinoin on hair growth in male mice. ISRN Pharmacol. 2014;2014:575423.
16. Rushton DH, Futterweit W, Kingsley D, et al. Quantitative assessment of spironolactone treatment in women with diffuse androgen-dependent alopecia. J Soc Cosmet Chem. 1991;42:317-25.
17. Schiavone G, Raskovic D, Greco J, et al. Platelet-rich plasma for androgenetic alopecia: a pilot study. Dermatol Surg. 2014 Sep;40(9):1010-9.
18. Leavitt M, Charles G, Heyman E, et al. HairMax LaserComb laser phototherapy device in the treatment of male androgenetic alopecia: a randomized, double-blind, sham device-controlled, multicentre trial. Clin Drug Investig. 2009;29(5):283-92.
19. Lanzafame RJ, Banche RR, Chiacchierini RP, et al. The growth of human scalp hair in females using visible red light laser and LED sources. Lasers Surg Med. 2014;46(8):601-7.
20. Munck A, Gavazzoni MF, Trüeb RM. Use of low-level laser therapy as monotherapy or concomitant therapy for male and female androgenetic alopecia. Int J Trichol. 2014;6(2):45-9.
21. Jimenez JJ, Wikramanayake TC, Bergfeld W, et al. Efficacy and safety of a low-level laser device in the treatment of male and female pattern hair loss: a multicenter, randomized, sham device-controlled, double-blind study. Am J Clin Dermatol. 2014;15(2): 115-27.
22. Kim H, Choi JW, Kim JY, et al. Low-level light therapy for androgenetic alopecia: a 24-week, randomized, double-blind, sham device-controlled multicenter trial. Dermatol Surg. 2013;39(8):1177-83.

CHAPTER

11

Future Trends in Hair Transplant Surgery

Carlos K Wesley

INTRODUCTION

Natural-appearing improvements in hair density and scalp coverage frequently achieved in hair restoration surgery (HRS) today have advanced in ways that barely resemble the initial attempts of J Dieffenbach and his contemporaries from the 1820s. Great strides have also been made in our field regarding perioperative patient comfort as well as heightening societal awareness of the success of hair transplantation. Building on our specialty's current foundation is inevitable. The specific direction in which our field will advance, however, invites speculation and imagination.

Hair transplantation has benefited from innovations in the form of both medical therapies and surgical devices. Innovation often requires outside financial investment, and the more recent advancements described herein may herald an overall increase in biotech venture capital dedicated to our specialty. Three favorable characteristics encourage outside investment in HRS as compared to other medical fields: (1) the method of physician reimbursement, (2) the regulatory restrictions, and (3) the intellectual property landscape. Most fields of medicine require physician reimbursement through restrictive insurance regulations, a practice that can delay pharmaceutical venture or thwart clinical adoption of a new biomedical device. Next, the relatively noninvasive nature of hair procedures often affords a Class I designation with the United States Food and Drug Administration (FDA). The classification of I versus the more stringent II or III can shave months or even years off the time required to realize a physician's promising idea. Finally, the relatively untapped frontier of intellectual property in our field invites creative investment. For example, a search on the United States Patent and Trademark Office website listing patents filed since 1976 reveals significantly more restrictive patent filings for skin (n = 291,959) and bone (n = 141,725) than claims on hair follicle (n = 2,935).

LOW-LEVEL LIGHT THERAPY

It was four decades after Dr Endre Mester's initial work suggesting lasers' stimulation of hair follicle growth in mice before the first laser received 510K FDA clearance to treat androgenetic alopecia (AGA) in 2007. Stimulating the shaved backs of mice with a ruby laser beam of 694 nm to elucidate any carcinogenic effects, this Hungarian physician instead discovered more rapid regrowth of murine hair.[1] Since that experiment, over 100 randomized and controlled studies have been performed, also confirming a photomodulating effect of low-level light therapy (LLLT). Nevertheless, a clear consensus regarding the efficacy and best clinical protocol of LLLT for hair growth has yet to emerge.

Biostimulation resulting from LLLT has been suggested to occur within the cellular mitochondria: specifically, targeting cytochrome c oxidase at the final stage of the electron transport system.[2] By relieving the inhibitory effect of nitric oxide (NO) on this chromophore (the photoacceptor that absorbs light photons), photons enable cytochrome c oxidase to perform cellular functions such as increasing adenosine triphosphate (ATP) production and transcription factor induction. These actions theoretically launch a cascade of cellular effects that stimulate anagen re-entry, prolong anagen phase duration, and halt premature catagen onset.[3]

One challenge in creating reproducible trials with LLLT is the large number of variables involved. Four parameters can be specified when performing LLLT: wavelength, irradiance, duration, and frequency of treatments. Wavelength determines the target tissue for absorption. Most commonly in human scalp, the photoacceptors are melanin, hemoglobin, and water. Low-level laser light ranges from wavelengths 500 to -1100 nm, within the spectrum of visible light. Irradiance is the power (W/cm^2) administered to a given area of treatment. A maximum irradiance of 0.005 W (or 5 mW) is allowed for LLLT devices in the United States.[2] The duration of irradiation is the energy (joules). The frequency, or the interval between therapies, also influences the level of cellular excitation by laser treatments and their clinical impact.

Low-level light therapy delivery can also be influenced by variables such as light transmission, type of beam, and distance from the treatment target. Human tissue can absorb, reflect, transmit, or scatter light. There can also be varying degrees of absorption based on the type of photoacceptor light encounters. For example, melanin in brown or black hair (eumelanin) has a much greater absorption tendency than blonde or red hair melanin (pheomelanin)—possibly influencing light transmission by 37%.[4,5] Patients with more hair volume, length, or curl may also have a markedly different amount of LLLT absorbed by the intended scalp tissue target than their less hirsute counterparts. Collimated (parallel columns) and coherent (parallel to one another with a constant phase difference and same frequency) beams of laser light are less divergent than those from light emitting diodes (LEDs) that are neither collimated nor coherent. While the more focused laser light beam may ensure 100% irradiance at a perpendicular angle to its target, the more divergent LED lights may cover a wider treatment area, but with a less predictable degree of reflection or irradiance. Finally, intensity of irradiation is inversely proportional to the square of the distance between the source and target ($I = 1/d^2$), thus providing another challenge to produce repeatable clinical outcomes.

In a LLLT study on hair, half of the 40 subjects were treated with a helmet-type LLLT product (LEDs of three different wavelengths: 630 nm, 650 nm, and 660 nm) or sham device for 18 minutes daily for 24 weeks. The treatment group demonstrated a significant improvement in mean changes of hair density and diameter ($p < 0.05$).[6] This indicated either a successful conversion of intermediate follicles to active terminal hairs or a triggering of resting telogen to active anagen hairs. However, subjective global assessment and subjective satisfaction between the LLLT-treated group and sham-treated population failed to achieve statistical significance.[6] A larger investigation involving 128 male and 141 female subjects was performed to evaluate three different models of the laser comb three times per week for 26 weeks (Figs. 11.1A and B).[7] This meta-analysis of four separate multicenter clinical trials was randomized, sham-controlled, and double-blinded. When results of all four studies were analyzed (two male and two female populations), a statistically significant increase in terminal hair density was observed for each group. The objective benefit of these microscopic findings, however, did not consistently predict patient satisfaction. Subjective questionnaires for self-assessment of overall improvement of hair loss condition (thickness/fullness) submitted by patients after 16 and 26 weeks of treatment reached statistical significance in only one of the two female populations investigated. Both male populations submitting self-evaluations failed to reach statistical significance regarding overall improvement.

While these clinical data show promise, LLLT involves high electricity consumption, at a relatively high cost (ranging from $695 to upward of $6075 for a laser instrument), and the need for eye protection. Furthermore, the biphasic nature of the dose response with LLLT has yet to be clearly elucidated. No tissue response occurs when the wavelength, irradiance, or duration is too low. Parameters set too high, however, can inhibit any tissue response. Interestingly, Dr Sharon Keene during her recent presentation on LLLT at the 2014 ISHRS Conference pointed out that cells in tissue culture demonstrate four peaks of deoxyribonucleic acid production when photostimulated by wavelengths of 614–624 nm, 668–684 nm, 751–772 nm, and 813–846 nm.[8] However, she also noted that none of the published literature on laser devices utilizes these wavelengths.[2] This inconsistency may represent a possible refinement or enhancement of LLLT in the future.

BIOENHANCED HAIR RESTORATION: SCALP MESOTHERAPY

Prostaglandin Analogs

Just as LLLT treatment for hair stemmed from a fortuitous observation, prostaglandin analogs for treating glaucoma were serendipitously found to increase eyelash growth.[9] Excitement continued to grow as animal studies corroborated the hypothesis that scalp hair would benefit similarly from this relatively simple mode of therapy. The success of murine scalp studies, however, has not yet translated into the same degree of human efficacy. Although a randomized, double-blind, placebo-controlled study of topical latanoprost 0.1% provided some evidence supporting the recruitment of vellus to terminal hair follicles, half of the 16 human subjects enrolled in this 24-week clinical trial demonstrated an equal or *worse* response to therapy than that observed in the placebo-injected portion of their scalp.[10]

In the future, perhaps just as the counterbalancing of prostaglandins provides harmony in human bronchial muscle tone (PGA2 increases contraction while PGE2 promotes relaxation), their opposing effects on hair may provide an important key to improving efficacy.[11] For example, PGD2 (which functionally inhibits hair lengthening and hair regeneration) is elevated in the bald scalp of men with AGA.[11] Scalp treatments such as bimatoprost and latanoprost that support follicle health may someday be effectively combined with those that downregulate the prostaglandins, which inhibit hair growth.

Platelet-Rich Plasma

Autologous platelet-rich plasma (PRP) injections into the scalp have become a popular nonsurgical procedure performed by physicians in our specialty. Meanwhile, it may also prove the least standardized method of treatment. At the 2013 ISHRS Conference, for instance, a panel of five well-respected HRS

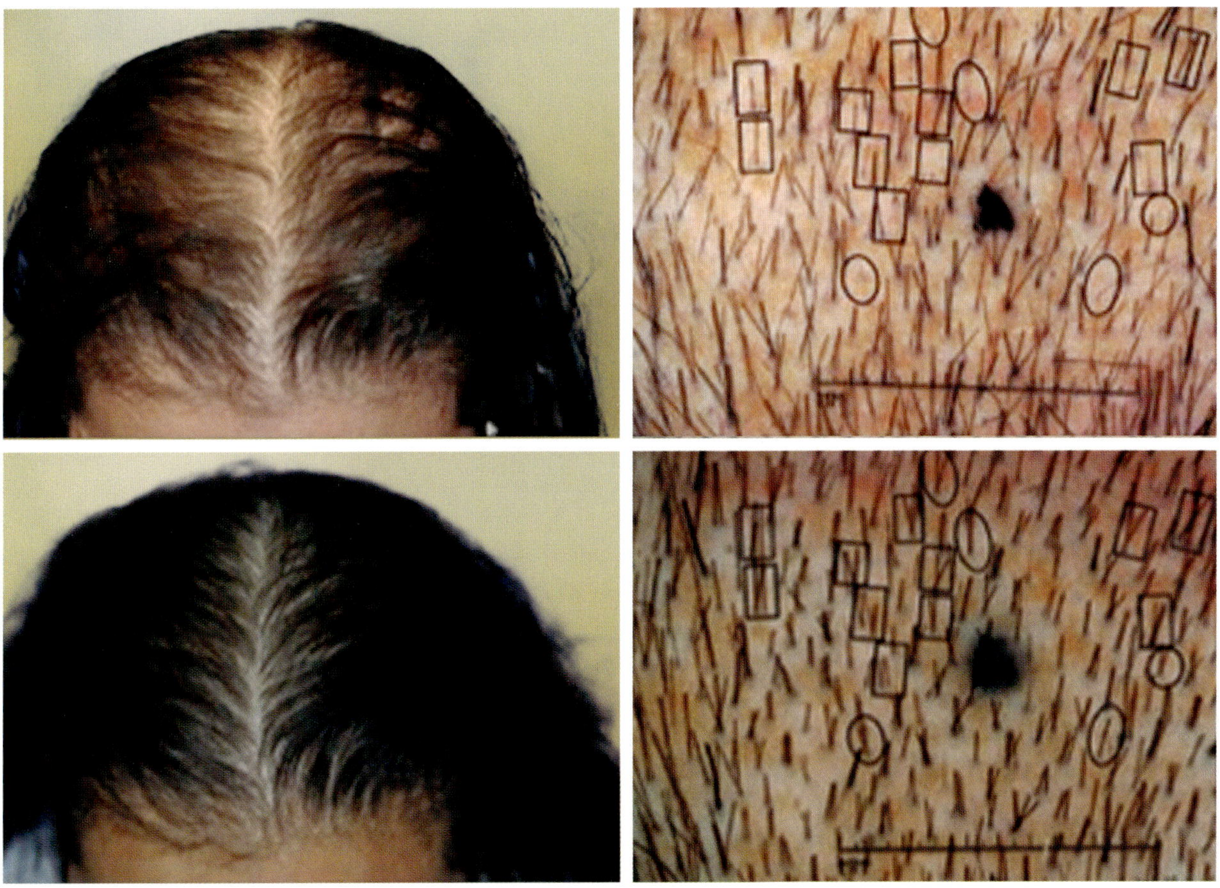

Fig. 11.1A: Androgenic alopecia before and after low-level light therapy treatment. Global photographs of a female patient before (a) and after (b) a 26-week treatment with a 12-beam laser comb. Magnified images of a male subject as seen before (c) and after (d) a 26-week treatment with a 9-beam laser comb. Ovals highlight follicle conversion from vellus to terminal hairs while rectangles indicate resting telogen to active anagen follicles.

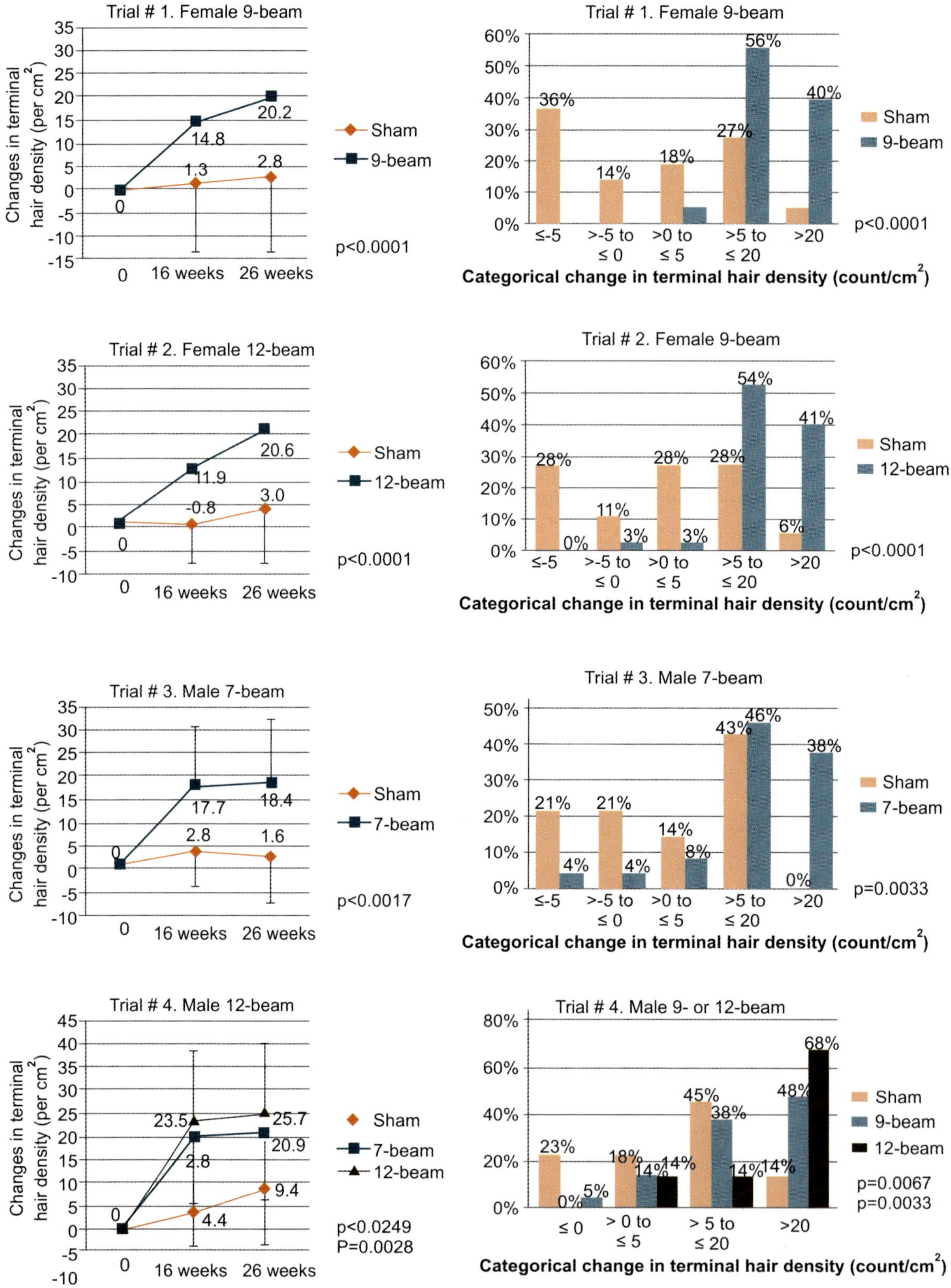

Fig. 11.1B: Both mean and categorical changes in density (counts per cm²) of terminal hair after treatment with either laser comb or sham device. P values are shown at 26 weeks. Bars reflect standard deviation.

Source: Permission and original image sought from Jimenez JJ, et al. Efficacy and safety of a low-level laser device in the treatment of male and female pattern hair loss: a multicenter, randomized, sham device-controlled, double-blind study. Am J Clin Dermatol. 2014;15(2):115-27.

practitioners was asked to describe their method of PRP isolation, concentration, interval of treatment, and results. All five responded differently to each criterion.

Platelet-rich plasma has numerous proposed mechanisms of action: (1) it stimulates proliferation and differentiation of follicular bulge area stem cells into follicle cells via upregulation of b-catenin; (2) it prolongs survival of dermal papilla (DP) cells by activating the protein kinase b (or AKT/PKB) and extracellular signal-related kinase signaling pathways; (3) it extends the anagen hair cycle phase by upregulating fibroblast growth factor 7; and (4) it increases vascular plexus surrounding follicles due to the release of platelet-derived growth factor and the secretion of vascular endothelial growth factor by the outer root sheath keratinocytes and DP fibroblasts.[12,13]

Although initial in vivo studies on mice showed promise, we presently lack firm clinical evidence that activated PRP can promote human hair growth. Li helped define signaling pathways and showed that subcutaneous injections of activated PRP in mice can increase DP cells and shorten the telogen-to-anagen transition.[13] These positive findings were further supported by Takikawa's observation that five intradermal injections of PRP performed at 2-to-3-week intervals in 26 co-ed human subjects generated a statistically significant increase both in hair diameter and perifollicular neovascularization.[14] Excitement surrounding these findings is tempered by other pilot studies demonstrating no clinical improvement in 80% of human patients ($n = 10$) after 6-week PRP treatments.[15] Even Khatu's recent clinical evidence of PRP's desirable conversion to a negative pull test after four scalp injections at 2-week intervals and Gentile's observed statistically significant increase in mean hair number and total hair density (number of hairs/cm^2) have been met with skepticism due to the relatively small and gender-limited nature of these human studies: 11 male subjects and 10 male subjects, respectively (Figs. 11.2A and B).[12,16] More large-scale investigations—such as a recent 64-patient observational study (42 men and 22 women) involving a two-injection approach at 3-month intervals—will help further elucidate the true efficacy of PRP in scalp therapy.[17] In this model, global physician assessment (GPA) scores for patient change were recorded by two evaluators using a macrophotographic protocol. Improvements in scalp hair coverage were observed in all subjects by one evaluator and in 62 of 64 by the other evaluator. In this study, patients appearing to benefit most from PRP injections suffered from a more severe baseline of AGA.

One significant limitation of scalp PRP mesotherapy is the questionable need for repeat treatments (Figs. 11.3A and B). Greco and Brandt observed a conversion of hair miniaturization back to terminal hair in nontransplanted follicles for up to 8 months after concentrated PRP scalp injections.[18] Treatment intervals vary greatly, however, in many subsequently published studies. Just as the optimal intervals of therapy have yet to be clearly defined, the ideal method of isolation also remains a source of debate. Due to disparate schools of thought regarding the value of leukocytes and fibrin content inclusion, four categories of PRP were defined by Dohan et al.[19] Pure platelet-rich plasma (P-PRP) contains a high concentration of platelets and a dearth of leukocytes. Leukocyte containing PRP includes harvesting of the buffy coat layer (enriched white cell population) as well as some residual erythrocytes. Pure platelet-rich fibrin is P-PRP mixed with an activator, such as a fibrin matrix, while leukocyte and platelet-rich fibrin involve no biochemical modification of the blood beside physical separation by centrifugation. Giusti et al. established the optimal platelet concentration of 1,500,000 platelets/μL with observations that lower or higher concentrations inhibited the desired angiogenic potential in human endothelial cells.[20] Some authors even suggest that optimal platelet concentrations should be individualized for each patient.[17]

Extracellular Matrices

In addition to the four categories of PRP listed above, this cellular milieu may be combined with other additives to enhance clinical outcomes. The incorporation of microparticles such as dalteparin and protamine has demonstrated positive influence on hair caliber.[14] The addition of extracellular matrices (ECMs) to autologous PRP therapy has also demonstrated benefit in both human and equine wound studies. It may prove to be a promising adjuvant to stimulate hair follicle cell proliferation or regeneration in the future.[21]

One ECM that is widely used in hair surgery is ACell MatriStem (ACell, Inc., Columbia, MD), derived from porcine urinary bladder matrix. Although expectations surrounding ACell have been dramatically

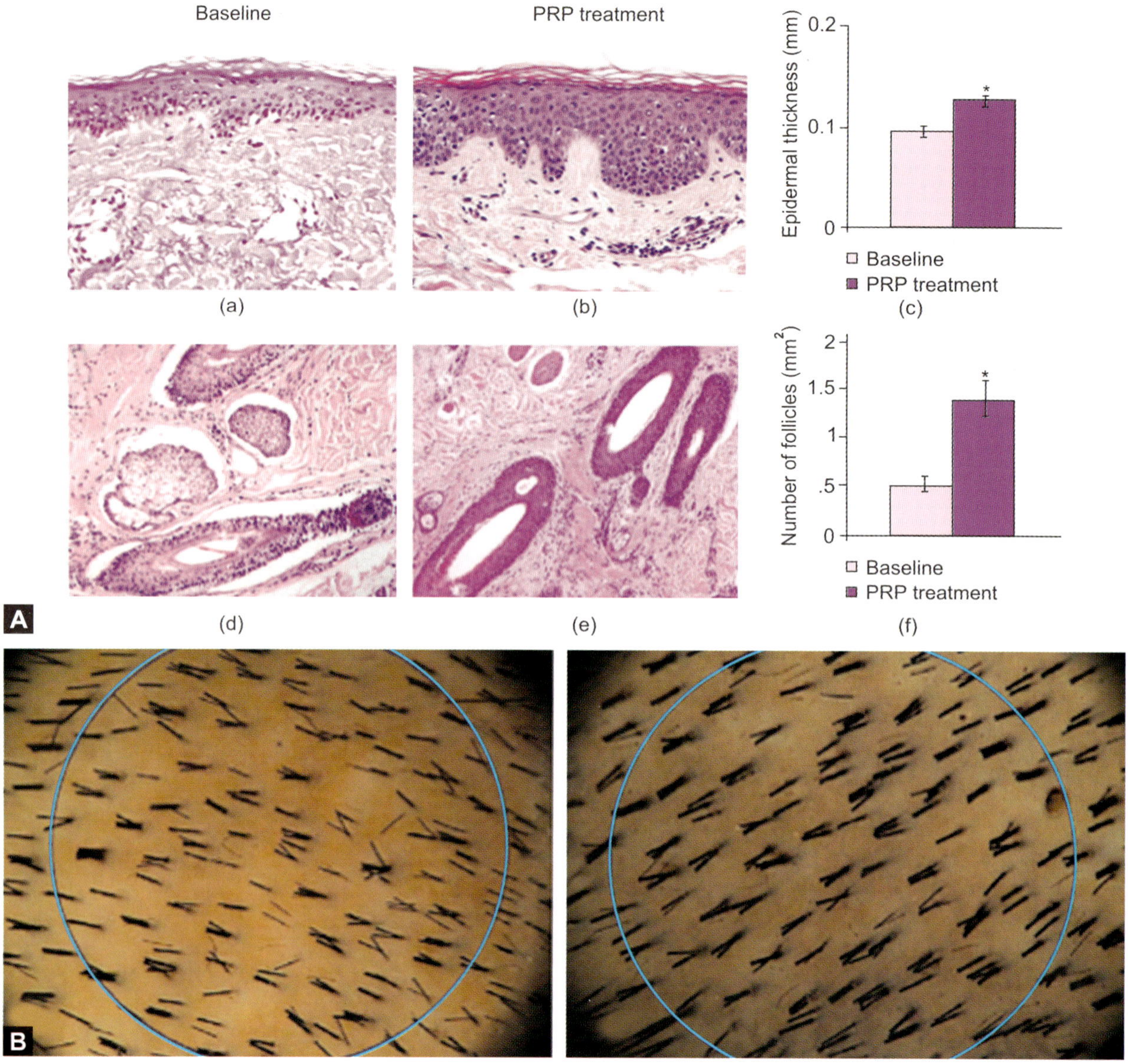

Figs. 11.2A and B: (A) Histologic images illustrating an increase in epidermal thickness before (a) and after (b) three platelet-rich plasma (PRP) treatments (mean 1,484,555 platelets/μL) at 1-month intervals. Dermal hair follicles also increase in number before (d) and after (e) the same series of PRP treatments. A bar graph representation of changes in epidermal thickness (c) and follicle number (f). (B) Changes in hair count and density as captured using a TrichoScan before (a) and after (b) the same PRP protocol.
Source: Permission and original image granted by Dr. P. Gentile for Cervelli V, et al. The effect of autologous activated platelet rich plasma (AA-PRP) injection on pattern hair loss: clinical and histomorphometric evaluation. Biomed Res Int. 2014;2014:760709.

tempered since the 2010 Press Release in which initial observation of transplanted "plucked" hair viability and regeneration was declared, its efficacy remains limited in HRS.[22] Anecdotal accounts of ACell's benefit have been published regarding (1) antifibrotic effects in follicular unit transplantation (FUT) strip healing, (2) tissue regenerative impact on follicular unit extraction (FUE) donor sites, and (3) angiogenic improvement as a graft coating product (Figs. 11.4A and B).[23] The dearth of evidence-based literature to match this popular regenerative product is staggering, however, as a Google search of "ACell MatriStem" and "hair" generates nearly 66,500 matches while the same term search on PubMed's list of peer-reviewed journal articles fails to yield a single result.

ROBOTIC TECHNOLOGY

Traditional donor ellipse harvesting remains the most commonly used technique worldwide (67.5%

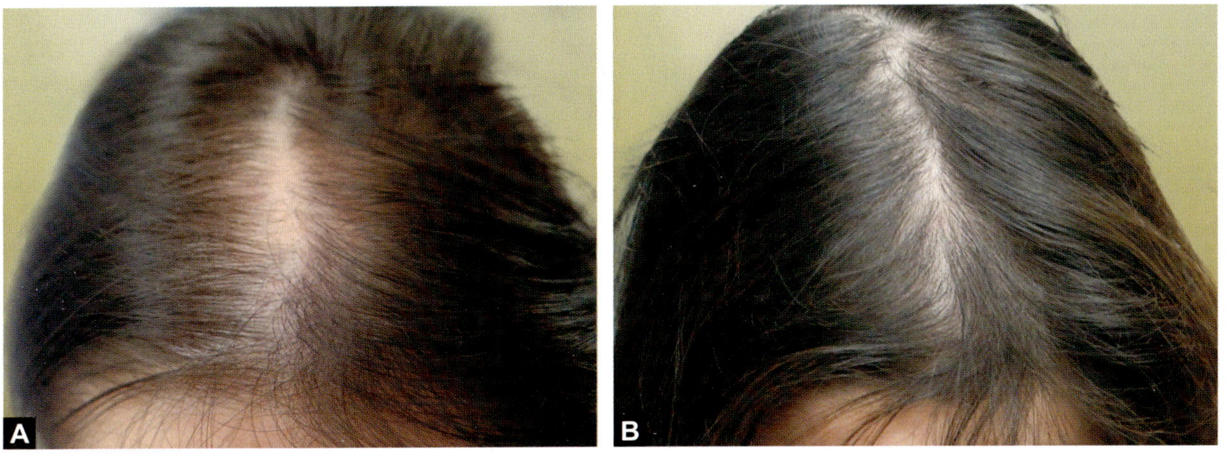

Figs. 11.3A and B: Global assessments of a 28-year-old biopsy-confirmed, female pattern hair loss sufferer at baseline (A) and 22 weeks after a single platelet-rich plasma (PRP) treatment (a double spin) combined with ACell Matristem powder (B). Debate exists surrounding the need for and frequency of repeat PRP treatments.
Courtesy: Carlos K. Wesley, MD.

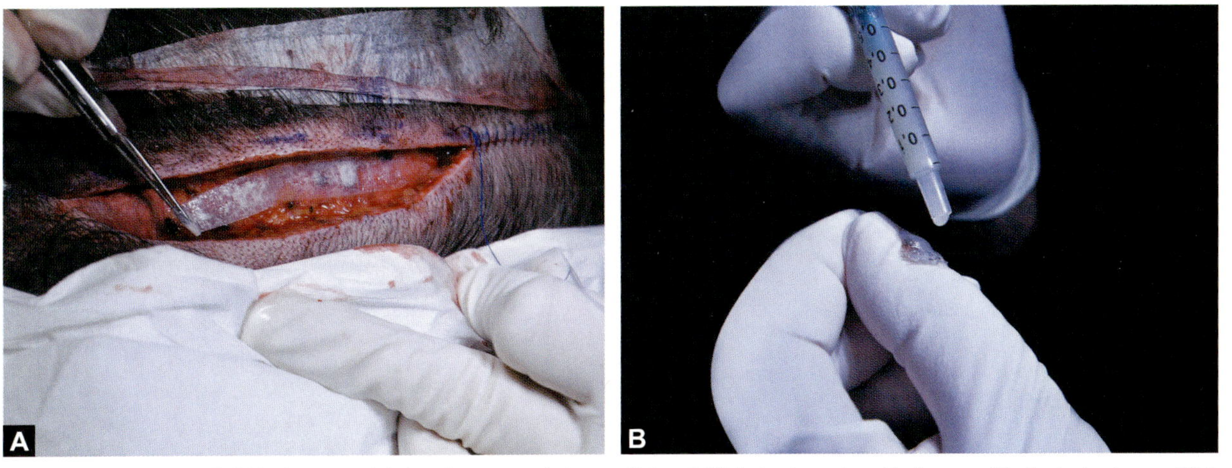

Figs. 11.4A and B: (A) ACell Matristem used during donor wound closure. Strips of ACell sheet are placed in the wound bed prior to closure. (B) A demonstration of a concentrated ACell suspension (powder dissolved in saline) placed onto follicular unit prior to implantation.
Source: Permission and original image sought from Dr Jerry Cooley.

vs 32.2% FUE performed in 2012). That being said, FUE has grown increasingly popular in recent years.[24] However, even with motorized punches, this technique can become extremely arduous when large 2000+ graft sessions are performed. The ARTAS robotic system (Restoration Robotics Inc., San Jose, CA) released in the fall of 2011 is a computer-assisted, interactive robotic FUE harvesting system that is controlled by the physician and designed to automate the process of FUE (Fig. 11.5).

The robot's concentrically arranged needle-in-needle FUE punch system contains a sharp bibeveled (inner) needle within a blunt outer punch.[25] After the initial 1-mm-diameter scoring incision with the inner needle, the scalp is dilated and dissected more deeply by the rotation and penetration of the blunt outer needle. Once the extraction process is eased by a suction system that elevates the targeted follicle, the graft is manually extracted by the operator. This process is made possible by stereocameras and a central image-processing system that measures and calculates the angle and direction of each target follicular unit (FU). Even incidental movements such as patient's breathing are detected and compensated for the robot's imaging feedback (Figs. 11.6A and B).

Although the robot typically determines the random targeting of follicles and rotations per minute, the physician can still control dissection parameters,

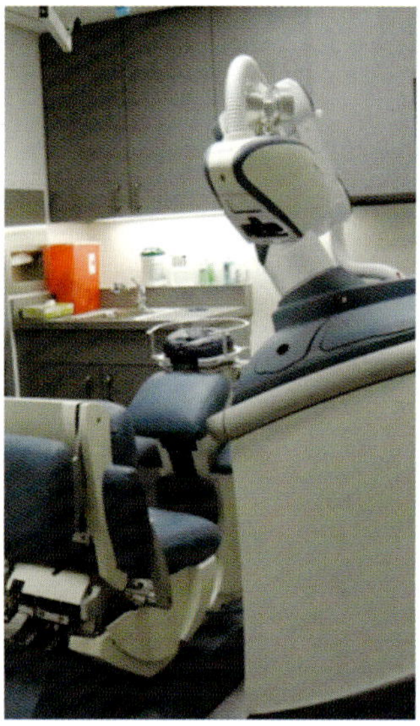

Fig. 11.5: The ARTAS Robotic-Assisted follicular unit extraction device.
Source: Permission and original image sought from Dr Marc Avram.

such as the harvesting density and the depth of punches (both inner and outer), and can even cherry-pick certain follicles to be extracted or passed over in manual mode. A noncontrolled, retrospective study of 22 Korean patients reported a viable graft yield of 95.1% and a transection rate of 4.9%.[25] The transection rate jumped to 29.2%, however, when 5-hair grafts were targeted—a compromise not normally seen in FUT. A more ethnically diverse population of 20 subjects (white, Asian, Middle Eastern, and Indian) resulted in an average transection rate of 6.6%.[26] Graft transection rates varied considerably from 0.4% to 32.1% with these mixed hair types. Meanwhile, published reports of FUT transection rates using experienced staff suggest a 1.59% graft transection rate.[26]

Makers of the ARTAS robotic system hope the device will eventually be able to create recipient

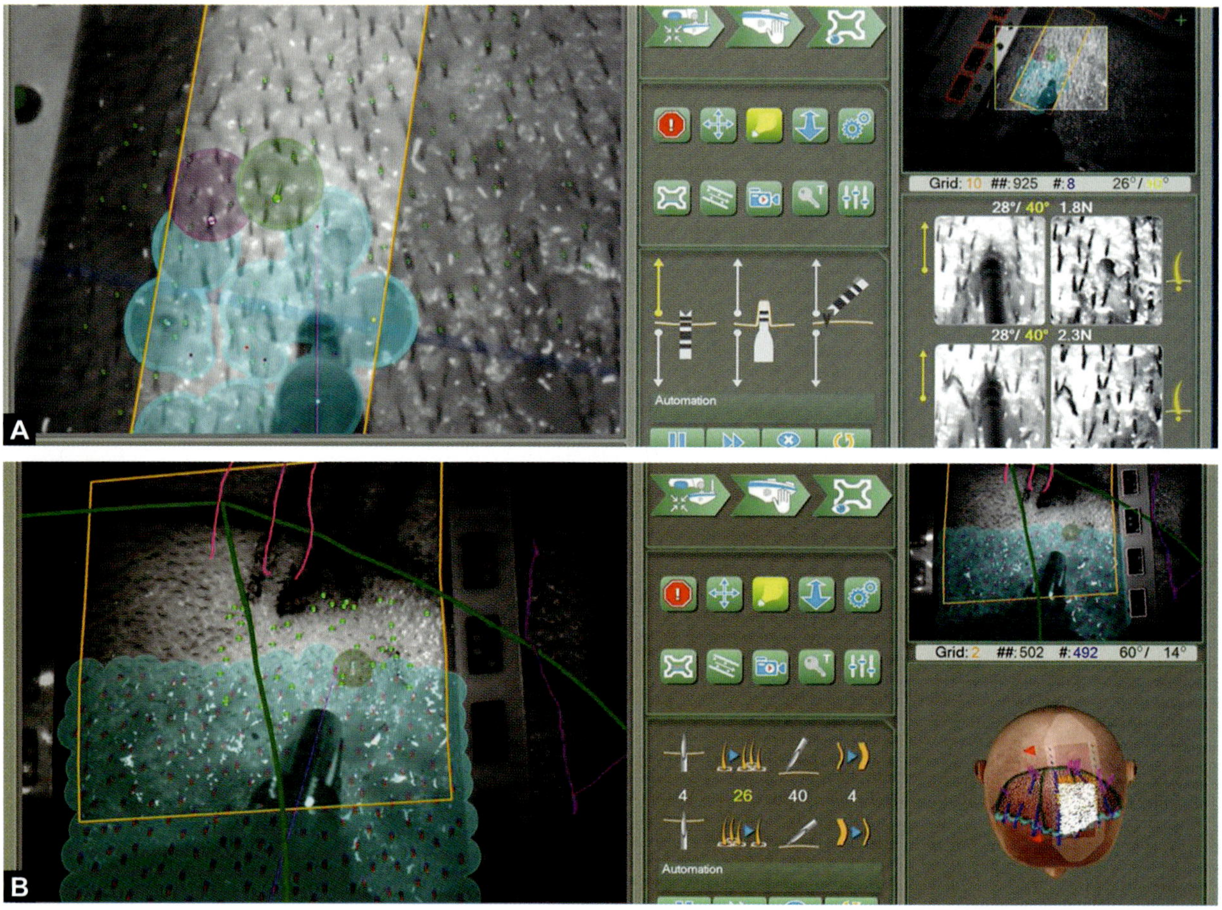

Figs. 11.6A and B: (A) Features of the ARTAS donor harvest display include the distribution and density of target follicles, depth of coring penetration, and a real-time image of each donor follicle punched. (B) The ARTAS recipient site creation display includes the ability to adjust the density, gauge, angle, direction, and overall pattern of incisions generated.
Courtesy: Photographs courtesy of Dr Miguel Canales.

sites and then place the grafts as well. The ARTAS Hair Studio software was designed to generate customized three-dimensional patient models based on standardized patient photographs, computerized calibration using interpupillary distance, and the physician's outlining of the recipient area.[27] In addition to specifying recipient site angle, direction, depth, average density, and total number of sites created, the operator can specify the avoidance or inclusion of pre-existing recipient hairs of a certain diameter. This last feature may enable physicians to avoid making incisions over large caliber existing hairs or previously transplanted hairs, thus ostensibly complementing existing density. Alternatively, miniaturized or vellus hair may be ignored or avoided on the basis of physician preference. In due course, this software will be able to simulate, prior to surgery, the actual post-transplant appearance of each candidate patient.

The disadvantages of robotic FUE harvesting and recipient site creation include the set-up time, the capital investment (in the United States, the ARTAS may cost over $265,000, depending on the product configuration), the need for a dedicated room for the large ARTAS system, and the requirement for shaving both the donor and recipient hairs to 1 mm in length.[25] Also, official ISHRS Comparison Between Strip Harvesting and FUE maintains that, "Grafts created with strip harvesting generally have a greater amount of surrounding tissue and fat". This may decrease the chance of dehydration and allow for greater leeway in manipulation of the grafts during placing and hence, better graft survival.[28] Until this denuded feature of FUE grafts is rectified, graft vulnerability may be best reduced by optimizing the manner in which FU are stored out of the body prior to subsequent implantation or by enhancing the postoperative scalp conditions into which follicles are transplanted.

HOLDING SOLUTIONS

Saline has been used for decades as a practical and inexpensive holding solution. Since then, many other agents have been introduced such as lactated ringers, various tissue culture media, and HypoThermosol (Biolife Solutions, Bothell, WA). The benefit of HypoThermosol (specifically designed for low temperature) is to prevent the intracellular influx of sodium and water into grafts, as well as to prevent ischemia reperfusion injury due to the glutathione and synthetic vitamin E it possesses.[29]

After Dr Jerry Cooley first observed marked intrapatient variability in scalp oxygen levels and responses to vasodilators as measured by visible light spectroscopy, he sought to provide a more supportive recipient environment in the scalp during the critical 5-day postoperative period during which grafts become revascularized in their new recipient tissue.[23] In 2005, Cooley tested the effects of ATP in HRS, initially as part of a graft holding solution and subsequently as a postoperative treatment for the grafts.[30] Liposomal ATP was first shown to protect ischemic cells in other organs (e.g. liver and heart) prior to its adoption in HRS.[31,32] Bioengineered ATPv contains two distinct forms of ATP: (1) the encapsulated ATP (intended as a 1:10 dilution of ATPv/graft holding solution) is designed to maintain intracellular ATP, while (2) the ATP in solution binds to cell surface receptors. Cooley's clinical observations support the theory that exogenous ATP help cells continue functioning while being stored out of the body. He has seen fewer cases of poor hair growth, better average results, and more exceptional results.[23] The debate regarding the ideal graft holding solution will continue and evolve with new supportive evidence.

PILOSCOPY

Perhaps even more important than protecting FUE-generated hair follicles in optimal storage solutions is preserving the protective tissue surrounding FUs. Chubby grafts represent the ideal in terms of this protective casing. Moreover, if the residual donor punctate scarring from FUE could be eliminated during the harvesting process of these "chubby" grafts, the two primary objectives of HRS would be met: to enhance survival of transplanted follicles while eliminating donor area scarring. Piloscopy is a novel subdermal approach to hair follicle harvesting that addresses both of these goals.

The piloscopic approach requires creation of a dissected cavity within the subcutaneous plane of the safe donor area (Figs. 11.7A to F).[33] A blunt dissection tool inserted through a 1.4-cm incision separates the dense connective tissue within this eventual plane. Through this single port (generally located just superior to the occipital protuberance), a working surgical cavity can be extended throughout the occipital and parietal zones of the safe donor area

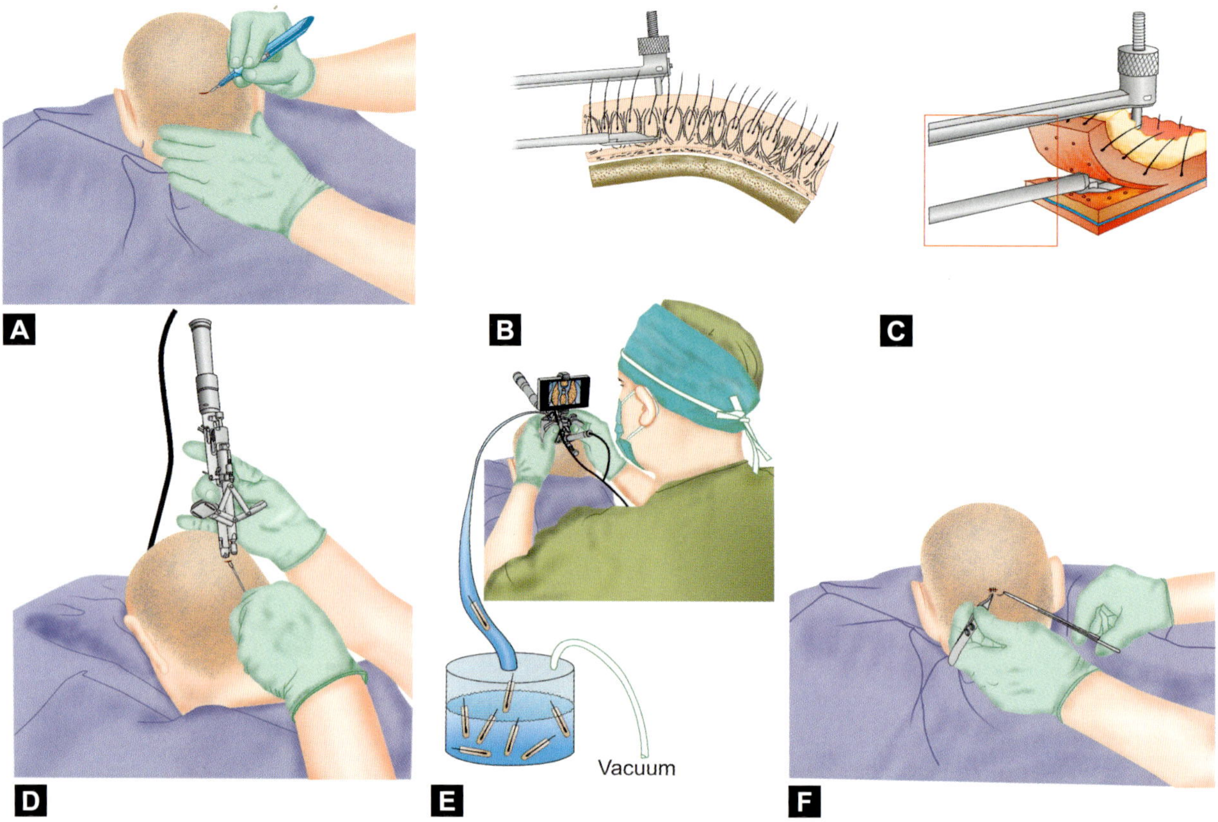

Figs. 11.7A to F: Steps involved in piloscopy. (A) A subdermal cavity within the dense subcutaneous layer of the scalp is created by introducing a piloscopic dissection device through a 1.4-cm port. A blunt dissection in the subdermal plane of the scalp (B and C) establishes the cavity. Only the subdermal arm in inserted through the port (D) and the external body of the piloscope, magnified monitor, and graft storage container rest outside of the patient's scalp (E). When the piloscopic harvest is complete, a single interrupted suture is applied to close the port of entry (F).
Source: Image previously submitted to Journal of Dermatologic Surgery (submitted).

(SDA). Throughout the procedure, the subdermal arm and the external body of the piloscope move in tandem (Fig. 11.8). The subdermal arm contains the apparatus capable of coring around stem-cell-enriched segments of the desired follicle (bulb and bulge) from a deep-to-superficial approach and cleaving off the shaft of the target follicle at its most superficial level. The physician, guided by a magnified image of the overlying portion of the desired follicle, aligns the target follicle before activating the cannula to core around and clip off the target follicle in a single motion while still maintaining the integrity of the overlying skin surface. A continuous sterile saline flush transports the extracted follicle into a graft storage chamber until its eventual implantation.

A double-blind, 16-month, six-patient clinical trial demonstrated that hair follicles harvested via the piloscopic approach (using a 1.2-mm piloscopic punch) produced no external evidence of trauma at the harvest sites and resulted in survival rates 45% greater than grafts harvested via traditional 1.0-mm punch FUE [$p < 0.001$].[34] A comparison of the intra-operative appearances of 1.0-mm FUE and 1.2-mm piloscopic harvesting methods can be viewed on a cadaveric scalp in Figures11.9A and B. Histologic and immunohistochemical assays using cytokeratin 15 (a biomarker for human epithelial follicular stem cells) also confirm CK15 activity within the bulge region of FU harvested piloscopically. Clinical subjects, while limited, have reported postoperative comfort and have not experienced telogen effluvium in the donor region after piloscopy.

While promising, considerable refinements in surgical instrumentation remain in order to achieve graft harvesting consistency and rates akin to current FUE standards. Still, theoretical benefits of piloscopy abound. Patients may not need to shave their head in order to benefit from this below-the-skin-surface approach. Curly-haired patients may no longer present the same ominous challenge they currently do as piloscopy's ability to shift the underlying portion of the follicle can standardize this unpredictable

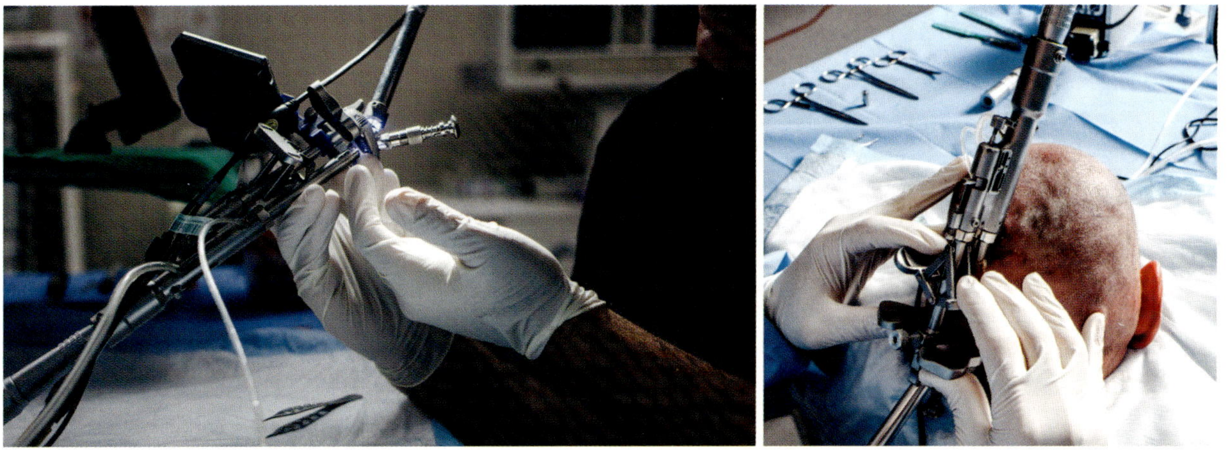

Fig. 11.8: The piloscopic surgical device. These images display the manner in which the piloscope is handled by the operator and the position upon the patient's scalp.
Courtesy: Photographs courtesy of Cole Wilson.

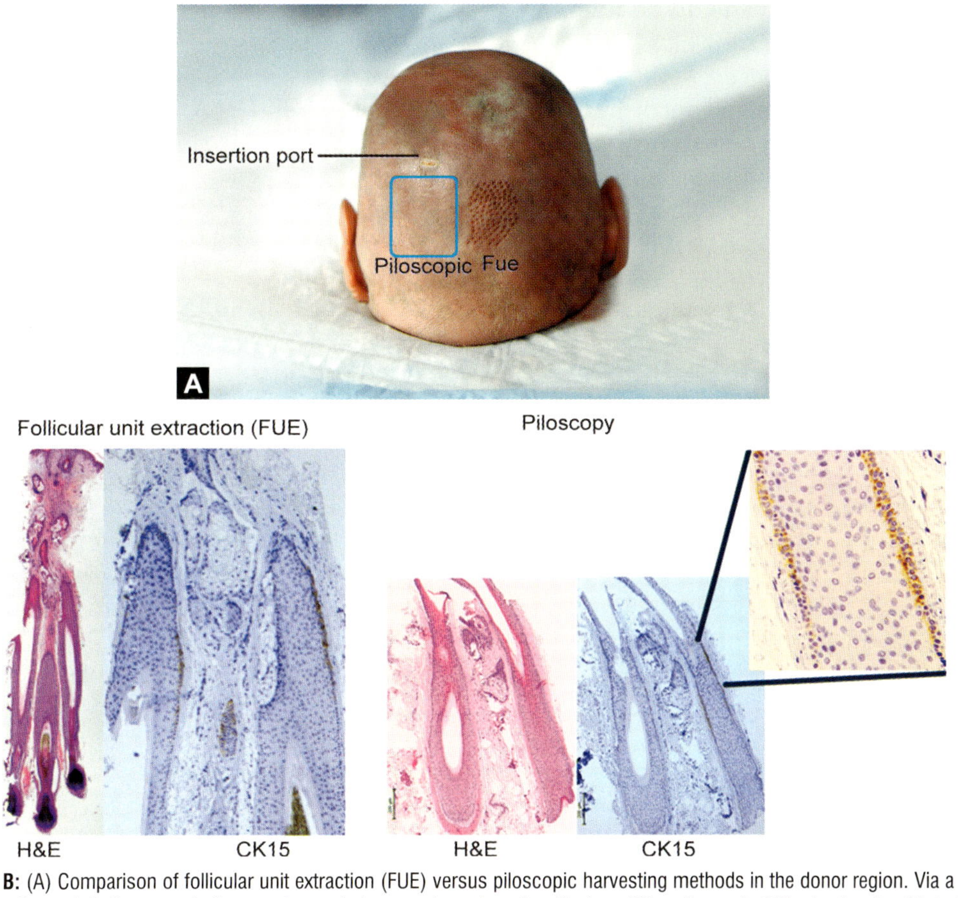

Figs. 11.9A and B: (A) Comparison of follicular unit extraction (FUE) versus piloscopic harvesting methods in the donor region. Via a 1.4-cm port of entry (labeled insertion point), the current piloscope harvested an equal number of grafts ($n = 98$) as those via FUE, at a density akin to that of adjacent FUE harvest and from the same size contralateral area of a cadaveric scalp. Evident in the regions from which FUs are harvested via the piloscopic approach is the well-maintained integrity of the overlying skin surface. (B) Hemoatoxilin–eosin and CK15 immunostaining of FUE and subdermal (i.e. piloscopic) grafts. CK15 stains stem cells at the bulge of FUE grafts (the cytoplasmic brown pigment at the peripheral later of the outer root sheath) (a). Piloscopic grafts also possess ample CK15 stained stem cells at the bulge region (b). However, unlike their FUE counterparts, the infundibulum and overlying skin surface are not present. These combined images indicate that piloscopic FU separation from overlying tissue is sufficiently superficial to include the stem-cell-enriched bulge during harvest with the current piloscopic device.
Source: Image previously submitted to Journal of Dermatologic Surgery (submitted).

variable. This same subdermal follicle manipulation can increase efficiency of the procedure, allowing multiple grafts to be harvested simultaneously *without* the epidermis—an anatomic benefit that enables immediate implantation. Finally, while the boundaries of the SDA should always be respected during a harvest in order to ensure prolonged survival of transplanted FU, any inadvertent piloscopic FU extraction beyond the anticipated SDA would be at least partially forgiven as piloscopy may eliminate the risk of leaving behind visible scarring. Further clinical investigations will confirm the efficacy, safety, and practicality of piloscopy in everyday clinical practice.

CELL THERAPY/CLONING

Hair follicle stem cells (HFSCs) are prime candidates for research in both hair restoration and many other fields of regenerative medicine. In addition to de novo generation of new hair follicles, HFSCs have furthered therapeutic perspectives for (1) healing of large, chronic leg ulcers; (2) treatment of third-degree burns; (3) and novel gene therapy strategies.[35] HFSCs originate from neuroectoderm cells during embryologic development, and are capable of forming new follicles and sebaceous glands as well as participating in the repair of the epidermis after injuries.[36,37]

Four general approaches to follicular neogenesis have been attempted. The first, implantation of dissociated cell cultures in which DP cells are isolated, multiplied in cell culture, and implanted, has not achieved success. RepliCel has focused their efforts toward a second method: implanting stimulating cells (e.g. cultured dermal sheath cup cells) that attach to existing miniaturized hairs in order to enhance their caliber. The two remaining methods involve implantation into recipient sites of bioengineered grafts that have begun follicular neogenesis in either culture dishes or an intermediate animal hosts.[38]

The reciprocal epithelial-mesenchymal interaction between epidermal stem cells (SCs) and mesenchymal SC in DP is essential in generating bioengineered grafts and achieving hair follicle neogenesis. Toyoshima illustrated orthotopic hair regeneration with implanted bioengineered hair follicle germ cells and Asakawa demonstrated ectopic bioengineered follicles transplanted via FUT in mice.[39,40] Hair produced in Asakawa's study possessed not only the correct anatomical structure, but also the proper connections with surrounding tissues and the ability to undergo repeated hair cycles. Yang et al.'s work transcended our believed limitation of the patient's hair follicle as the finite source for regenerative cells by demonstrating that somatic (normal body) cells induced into pluripotent stem cells can then be transformed into epithelial stem cells capable of producing all human hair follicle epithelial layers.[41] These newly generated cells produced intact hair follicles when combined with dermal cells and injected into immunodeficient mice.

While these fresh, new findings certainly prove encouraging, it has actually been over 40 years since rodent DP cells were first observed to induce de novo follicle growth after transplantation into recipient murine skin.[42] The consistency of results in murine models, however, has failed to translate into human subjects to the same degree. Even more discouraging was discovering how quickly human hair SC begin to lose their full regenerative potential. For when human DP cells were removed from their hair follicle microenvironment and grown in culture, they immediately lost contextual and positional cues from surrounding epithelial cells.[43]

This discouraging finding, however, sparked a new perspective and approach to human hair cell therapy by Higgins et al. that led to an exciting result. Higgins et al. hypothesized that the first step in successful hair neogenesis in humans is promoting cultured human DP cells to undergo self-aggregation. Interestingly, a striking difference occurs when DP cells are injected into the skin of rodents versus humans: whereas DP cells aggregate in murine models, they dissipate in human scalp.[43] Of the complex array of gene expressions involved in regulating HFSC, the Wnt/ß-catenin and BMP/TGF-ß signaling pathways are considered the most essential.[44] Using global microarray profiling, very rapid and profound molecular signature changes were observed in these specific pathways with the 3D (aggregated) to two-dimensional (2D; dissipated) conversion (Fig. 11.10). These changes were theorized to account for the rapid loss of human DP's capacity for hair follicle induction. Using 3D spheroids rather than traditional 2D Petri dishes to culture human DP cells and subsequently injecting the 3D spheroid cultures between the epidermis and dermis of human foreskin tissue, de novo hair follicles formed in five of seven donors 6-week post-transplantation (Figs. 11.11A to C).[43] Although this method elicited new follicle formation in recipient human skin, sebaceous glands were not

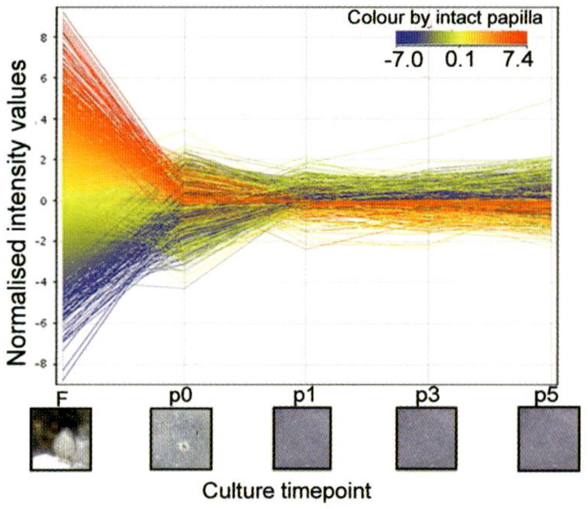

Fig. 11.10: Global microarray profiling demonstrates rapid loss of dermal papilla transcription factor activity with each in vivo passage on a two-dimensional Petri dish (e.g. p0, p1, etc.). Of note, expressions specific to the Wnt/ß-catenin and BMP/TGF-ß signaling pathways declined rapidly. These are considered by many most essential factors in follicular neogenesis.
Source: Permission and original image sought from Higgins CA, et al. Microenvironmental reprogramming by three-dimensional culture enables dermal papilla cells to induce de novo human hair-follicle growth. Proc Natl Acad Sci USA. 2013;110(49):19679-88.

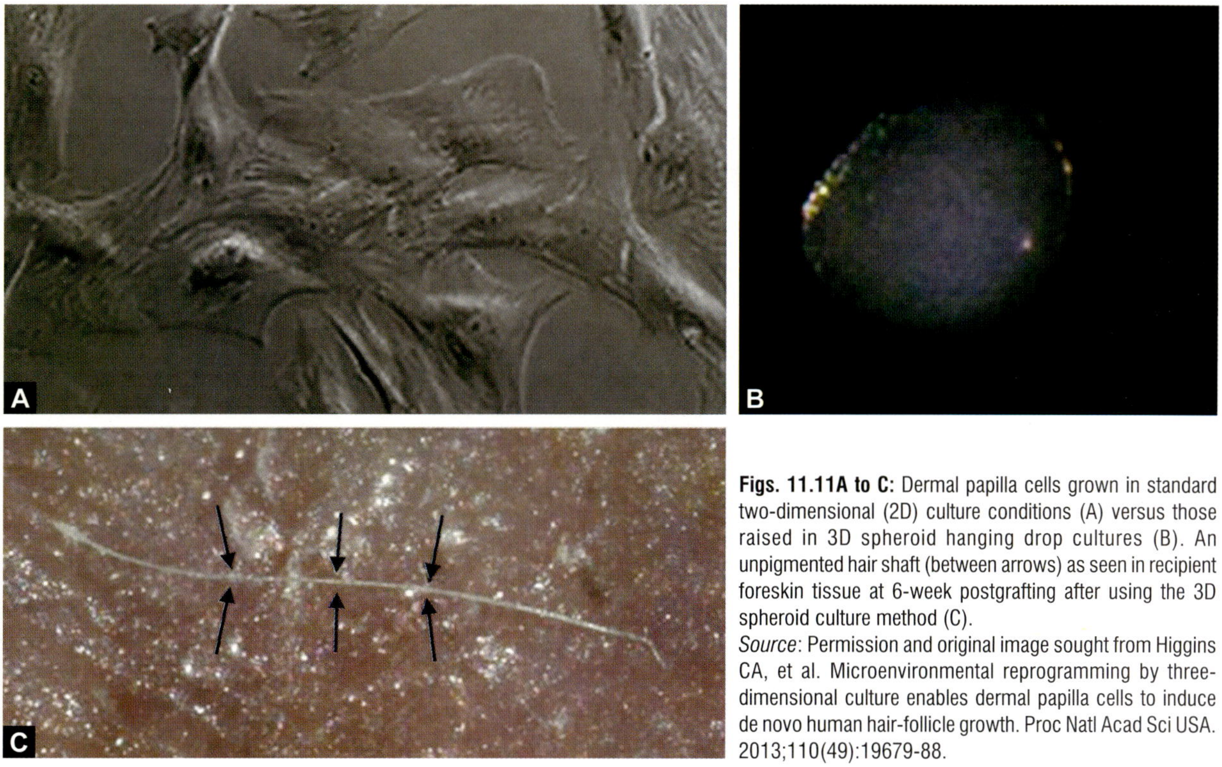

Figs. 11.11A to C: Dermal papilla cells grown in standard two-dimensional (2D) culture conditions (A) versus those raised in 3D spheroid hanging drop cultures (B). An unpigmented hair shaft (between arrows) as seen in recipient foreskin tissue at 6-week postgrafting after using the 3D spheroid culture method (C).
Source: Permission and original image sought from Higgins CA, et al. Microenvironmental reprogramming by three-dimensional culture enables dermal papilla cells to induce de novo human hair-follicle growth. Proc Natl Acad Sci USA. 2013;110(49):19679-88.

seen, the follicles that grew were small, and de novo growth often failed to produce hair fibers that exited the skin surface.

Although fully functional follicle generation de novo will require more than just physical manipulation of cultured DPs from 2D to 3D, this represents a step toward successful hair cell therapy. Nonautonomous communication with neighboring cells in the follicle microenvironment may prove critical in further advancing human hair neogenesis.

CONCLUSION

Perhaps some of the influential neighboring cells were highlighted in Dr Rodney Sinclair's fascinating feature presentation at the 2014 ISHRS conference on the arrector pilli muscle's possible influence on individual FU's development and ultimate regression throughout a human lifetime.[45] Until all elusive links between the numerous pathways are fully elucidated and legitimate concerns surrounding cell therapy's unregulated cell growth leading to tumor formation are allayed, we as a field will benefit from the continuous process of discovery.

REFERENCES

1. Hamblin MR. Mechanisms of laser-induced hair regrowth. Dose-Response (Prepress) Formerly Nonlinearity in Biology, Toxicology, and Medicine, University of Massachusetts. 2009.
2. Keene SA. The science of light biostimulation and low level laser therapy (LLLT). Hair Transplant Forum Int. 2014;24(6):204-9.
3. Avci P, Gupta GK, Clark J, et al. Low-level laser (light) therapy (LLLT) for treatment of hair loss. Lasers Surg Med. 2013;9999:1.
4. Steiner R. Laser tissue interactions. In: Raulin C, Karsai S (Eds). Laser and IPL Technology in Dermatology and Aesthetic Medicine. Berlin: Springer; 2011. pp. 23-36.
5. Mustafa FH, Jaafar MS, Ismail A. Influence of hair color in photodynamic dose activation in PDT for scalp disease. In: Abu Osman NA, Wan Abas WAB, Abdul Wahab AK, Ting HN (Eds). IFMBE Proceedings, Vol. 35. Berlin: Springer; 2011.
6. Kim H, Choi JW, Kim JY, et al. Low-level light therapy for androgenetic alopecia: a 24-week, randomized, double-blind, sham device-controlled multicenter trial. Dermatol Surg. 2013; 39:1177-83.
7. Jimenez JJ, Wikramanayake TC, Bergfeld W, et al. Efficacy and safety of a low-level laser device in the treatment of male and female pattern hair loss: a multicenter, randomized, sham device-controlled, double-blind study. Am J Clin Dermatol. 2014;15 (2):115-27.
8. Keene SA. Low level laser therapy (LLLT): How Does it Work? What is the difference between the different devices? Lecture ISHRS 22nd Annual Scientific Meeting. Kuala Lumpus, Malaysia, October 9, 2014.
9. Johnstone MA, Albert DM. Prostaglandin-induced hair growth. Surv Ophthalmol. 2002;47:S185-202.
10. Blume-Peytavi U. A randomized double-blind placebo-controlled pilot study to assess the efficacy of a 24-week topical treatment by latanoprost 0.1% on hair growth and pigmentation in healthy volunteers with androgenetic alopecia. J Am Acad Dermatol. 2012;66(5):794-800.
11. Nieves A, Garza LA. Does prostaglandin D2 hold the cure to male pattern baldness? Exp Dermatol. 2014;23(4):224-7.
12. Cervelli V, Garcovich S, Bielli A, et al. The effect of autologous activated platelet rich plasma (AA-PRP) injection on pattern hair loss: clinical and histomorphometric evaluation. Biomed Res Int. 2014;2014: 760709.
13. Li ZJ, Choi HI, Choi DK, et al. Autologous platelet-rich plasma: a potential therapeutic tool for promoting hair growth. Dermatol Surg. 2012;38:1040-46.
14. Takikawa M, Nakamura S, Ishirara M, et al. Enhanced effect of platelet-rich plasma containing a new carrier on hair growth. Dermatol Surg. 2011;37:1721-9.
15. Marwah M, Godse K, Patil S, et al. Is there sufficient research data to use platelet-rich plasma in dermatology? Int J Trichology. 2014;6(1):35-6.
16. Khatu SS, More YE, Gokhale NR, et al. Platelet-rich plasma in androgenic alopecia: myth or an effective tool. J Cutan Aesthet Surg. 2014;7(2):107-10.
17. Schiavone G, Raskovic D, Greco J, et al. Platelet-rich plasma for androgenetic alopecia: a pilot study. Dermatol Surg. 2014;40:1010-19.
18. Greco J, Brandt R. The effects of autologous platelet rich plasma and various growth factors on non-transplanted miniaturized hair. Hair Transplant Forum Int. 2009;19(2):49-50.
19. Dohan EDM, Ramusson L, Albrektsson T. Classification of platelet concentrates: from pure platelet rich plasma (P-PRP) to leucocyte-and-platelet-rich fibrin (L-PRF). Trends Biotechnol. 2009;27:158-67.
20. Giusti I, Rughetti A, D'Ascenzo S, et al. Identification of an optimal concentration of platelet gel for promoting angiogenesis in human endothelial cells. Transfusion. 2009;49: 771-8.
21. Clark RA. Synergistic signaling from extracellular matrix-growth factor complexes. J Invest Dermatol. 2008;128:1354-5.
22. Hitzig G. Researchers develop first successful hair cloning technique—major advancement in hair restoration. Available from PR.com. Denver, NC: LA Management Co.; Jan 06, 2010.
23. Cooley JE. Bio-enhanced hair restoration. Hair Transplant Forum Intl. 2014;24(4):127-30.
24. International Society of Hair Restoration Surgery: 2013 Practice Census Results. 2013: 11.
25. Shin JW, Kwon SH, Kim SA, et. al. Characteristics of robotically harvested hair follicles in Koreans. J Am Acad Dermatol. 2015; 72(1):146-50.
26. Avram MR, Watkins SA. Robotic follicular unit extraction in hair transplantation. Dermatol Surg. 2014; 40:1319-27.
27. Bernstein RM, Wolfeld MB, Zingaretti G. Robotic recipient site creation in hair transplantation. Hair Transplant Fourm Intl. 2014;24(3):95-7.
28. International Society of Hair Restoration Surgery. Comparison between strip harvesting and follicular unit extraction: a fair and balanced view. [online] www.ishrs.org. Aug. 1, 2010.
29. Mathew A. A review of cellular biopreservation considerations during hair transplantation. Hair Transplant Forum Intl. 2013;23(1):1,7-11.
30. Ehringer W. Letter to the Editor Re: Dr Jerry Cooley's "Bio-enhanced hair restoration." Hair Transplant Forum Intl. 2014;24(4):195.
31. Korb V, Tep K, Escriou V, et al. Current data on ATP-containing liposomes and potential prospects to enhance cellular energy status for hepatic applications. Crit Rev Ther Drug Carrier Syst. 2008; 25(4):305-45.

32. Hartner WC, Verma DD, Levchenko TS, et al. ATP loaded liposomes for treatment of myocardial ischemia. Wiley Interdiscip Rev Nanomed Nanobiotechnol. 2009;1(5):530-9.
33. Wesley CK. Piloscopy. In: Lam S, Williams K, Karamanovski E (Eds). Hair Transplant 360°. Vol. 4. Philadelphia: Jaypee Brothers (in press).
34. Wesley CK, Poblet E, Jimenez F. A novel subdermal approach to harvest intact hair follicles maintains transplanted graft viability without evidence of donor scarring. Dermatol Surg. (submitted).
35. Tiede S, Kloepper JE, Bodo E, et al. Hair follicle stem cells: walking the maze. Eur J Cell Biol. 2007;82(7); 355-76.
36. Fuchs E. Scratching the surface of skin development. Nature. 2007;445(7130): 834-42.
37. Yang L, Peng R. Unveiling hair follicle stem cells. Stem Cell Rev. 2010;6(4):658-64.
38. Cooley JE. Hair sciences: a review of follicular cell implantation and stem cell hair regrowth. [online] Available from ISHRS.org [Accessed May, 2014].
39. Asakawa K, Toyoshima KE, Ishibashi N, et al. Hair organ regeneration via the bioengineered hair follicular unit transplantation. Sci Rep. 2012;2:424.
40. Toyoshima KE, Asakawa K, Ishibashi N, et al. Fully-functional hair follicle regeneration through the rearrangement of stem cells and their niches. Nat Commun. 2012;3:784.
41. Yang R, Zheng Y, Burrows M, et al. Generation of folliculogenic human epithelial stem cells from induced pluripotent stem cells. Nat Commun. 2014; 5:3071.
42. Oliver RF. The induction of hair follicle formation in the adult hooded rat by vibrissa dermal papillae. J Embryol Exp Morphol. 1970;23(1): 219-36.
43. Higgins CA, Chen JC, Cerise JE, et al. Microenvironmental reprogramming by three-dimensional culture enables dermal papilla cells to induce de novo human hair-follicle growth. Proc Natl Acad Sci USA. 2013;110(49):19679-88.
44. Mokos AB, Mosler AL. Advances in a rapidly emerging field of hair follicle stem cell research. Coll Antropol. 2014:38(1);373-8.
45. Sinclair R. "Androgenetic Alopecia: The New Insight into the Role of Arrector Pili Muscle in Hair Biology." Lecture ISHRS 22nd Annual Scientific Meeting in Kuala Lumpur, Malaysia, Oct 9, 2014.

Index

Note: Page numbers followed by *f* and *t* indicate figures and tables, respectively.